B.C.

PSYCHOSOCIAL ISSUES
in
MALIGNANT DISEASE

Titles of related interest

GROSS   Oncogenic Viruses

MATHE & REIZENTSEIN   Pathophysiological Aspects of Cancer Epidemiology

WATSON & MORRIS   Psychological Aspects of Cancer

PSYCHOSOCIAL ISSUES

in

MALIGNANT DISEASE

Proceedings of the First Annual Conference
Organized by the British Psychosocial Oncology Group
London, 7–8 November 1984

Edited by

M. WATSON

and

S. GREER

Faith Courtauld Unit, King's College, London, UK

PERGAMON PRESS

OXFORD • NEW YORK • TORONTO • SYDNEY • FRANKFURT

U.K.	Pergamon Press Ltd., Headington Hill Hall, Oxford OX3 0BW, England
U.S.A.	Pergamon Press Inc., Maxwell House, Fairview Park, Elmsford, New York 10523, U.S.A.
CANADA	Pergamon Press Canada Ltd., Suite 104, 150 Consumers Road, Willowdale, Ontario M2J 1P9, Canada
AUSTRALIA	Pergamon Press (Aust.) Pty. Ltd., P.O. Box 544, Potts Point, N.S.W. 2011, Australia
FEDERAL REPUBLIC OF GERMANY	Pergamon Press GmbH, Hammerweg 6, D-6242 Kronberg, Federal Republic of Germany
JAPAN	Pergamon Press Ltd., 8th Floor, Matsuoka Central Building, 1-7-1 Nishishinjuku, Shinjuku-ku, Tokyo 160, Japan
BRAZIL	Pergamon Editora Ltda., Rua Eça de Queiros, 346, CEP 04011, São Paulo, Brazil
PEOPLE'S REPUBLIC OF CHINA	Pergamon Press, Qianmen Hotel, Beijing, People's Republic of China

First edition 1986

Library of Congress Cataloguing in Publication Data
Psychosocial issues in malignant disease.
1. Cancer—Psychological aspects—Congresses.
2. Cancer—Social aspects—Congresses.
I. Watson, M.
II. Greer, S. (Steven).
III. British Psychosocial Oncology Group.
[DNLM: 1. Neoplasms—psychology—congresses. QZ 200 P9755 1984]
RC262.P785 1985 616.99'4'0019 85-26043
British Library Cataloguing in Publication Data
British Psychosocial Oncology Group. *Conference (1st: 1984: London)*
Psychosocial issues in malignant disease.
1. Cancer—Psychological aspects.
2. Cancer—Social aspects.
I. Title.
II. Watson, Margaret, 1947–.
III. Greer, S.
616.99'4'0019 RC262
ISBN 0 08 032010 4

Printed in Great Britain by A. Wheaton & Co. Ltd., Exeter

Preface

In this book the proceedings of the first meeting of the British Psychosocial Oncology Group are reported. The desire for a multi-disciplinary forum led to the formation of this new professional association in November 1983. Our aim is to encourage collaborative interdisciplinary studies of patients with cancers, in order to extend and deepen the understanding of both the cancer process and of the individuals who develop these diseases.

A beginning has been made in this area, as attested by the papers presented at this meeting and by the small, but growing, scientific literature on the psychosocial aspects of cancer. In the first section of this volume reports on support and therapeutic programmes are presented which aim to alleviate the distress associated with the diagnosis and treatment of cancer. Section Two covers a number of important issues ranging from the problems surgeons face when dealing with cancer patients, the measurement of psychological morbidity and the importance, to some patients, of contact with fellow cancer sufferers. Section Three contains papers which help to clarify the extent of the problems and degree of distress which some patients experience as a result of the diagnosis and treatment of cancer.

Maggie Watson
Steven Greer

Acknowledgements

We would like to thank the following for their contributions to this meeting: Dame Cicely Saunders, for a stimulating inaugural address; Dr. Keith Pettingale, Mr. John Anderson and Professor Tim McElwain who kindly acted as chairmen of the conference sessions; Dr. Peter Maguire and Dr. Grace Christ for their informative presentations; the Bursar of Normanby College for allowing the use of the Wolfson Lecture Theatre; and finally Maria Wong, secretary of the Faith Courtauld Unit, for the major contribution she made to the organization of the conference.

Contents

List of Contributors

ASHCROFT, J. J.	Sub-department of Clinical Psychology, New Medical School, University of Liverpool, U.K.
BINDEMANN, S.	Department of Clinical Oncology, Gartnavel General Hospital, Glasgow, U.K.
VAN DEN BORNE, H. W.	Institute for Social Scientific Research, University of Tilburg, The Netherlands.
CALMAN, K. C.	Department of Clinical Oncology, Gartnavel General Hospital, Glasgow, U.K.
DEVLEN, J.	Department of Psychiatry, University Hospital of South Manchester, U.K.
HABESHAW, T.	Department of Clinical Oncology, Gartnavel General Hospital, Glasgow, U.K.
HOPWOOD, P.	Department of Psychiatry, University Hospital of South Manchester, U.K.
HUGHES, J. E.	Royal South Hants Hospital, Southampton, U.K.
KAYE, S. B.	Department of Clinical Oncology, Gartnavel General Hospital, Glasgow, U.K.
LANSDOWN, R. G.	The Hospital for Sick Children, Great Ormond Street, London, U.K.
LEINSTER, S. J.	Department of Surgery, Royal Liverpool Hospital, U.K.
LUNT, B. J.	Department of Community Medicine, Southampton General Hospital, U.K.
MILSTED, R. A. V.	Department of Clinical Oncology, Gartnavel General Hospital, Glasgow, U.K.
MORRIS, T.	Faith Courtauld Unit, King's College School of Medicine and Dentistry, London, U.K.
PRUYN, J. F. A.	Institute for Social Scientific Research, University of Tilburg, The Netherlands.
RAY, C.	Department of Psychology, Brunel University, Uxbridge, U.K.

SLADE, P. D.	Sub-department of Clinical Psychology, New Medical School, University of Liverpool, U.K.
STRINGER, P.	Social Psychology Department, University of Nijmegen, The Netherlands.
WATSON, M.	Faith Courtauld Unit, King's College School of Medicine and Dentistry, London, U.K.
WELSH, J.	Department of Clinical Oncology, Gartnavel General Hospital, Glasgow, U.K.

SECTION ONE

Support Programmes and Therapeutic Methods

Enhancement of Quality of Life with Relaxation Training in Cancer Patients Attending a Chemotherapy Unit

S. BINDEMANN, R. A. V. MILSTED, S. B. KAYE,
J. WELSH, T. HABESHAW and K. C. CALMAN

ABSTRACT

One hundred and nineteen patients undergoing treatment for various malignancies in a hospital oncology unit developed psychologic problems which were unrelieved by anxiolytic or anti-depressant-type drugs. All except seven patients were offered relaxation training (ReT), comprising simple breathing exercises, progressive muscle relaxation (PMR) and hypnosis. Sixty-eight patients agreed to participate and after initial training continued to induce profound relaxation by means of an audio tape-recording. Progress was reviewed at prescribed intervals, and qualitative changes in "psychologic", "social" and "other behavioural" criteria were assessed by the patients, their immediate relatives and by members of oncology medical and nursing staff. Concordance in such levels of assessment was high. In all, fourteen patients failed to participate until completion of the study. Of this number, five male and five female patients died, whilst the remainder defaulted from the study. One male patient and two female patients claimed not to have benefited at all. Reported and observed benefits of ReT indicated marked improvement in quality of life, including improved psychologic and social functioning, with concomitant reduction of analgesic and/or psychotropic drug intake. Some patients reported an enhanced capacity to tolerate further chemotherapy. Relaxation training appeared to make a valuable contribution to terminal care.

Difficulty in distinguishing between appropriate unhappiness and pathological anxiety or depression in the cancer patient is well known. Diagnosis of malignancy is in itself likely to elicit a stressful response, especially from the informed patient. Such a state of affairs is frequently exacerbated by the noxious side-effects of necessarily aggressive anti-cancer treatments.[1]* However, failure

* Superscript numbers refer to References at the end of the article.

3

to recognize the possible implications for psychopathology can lead to the development of chronic emotional and behavioural dysfunction.[2] This undoubtedly impairs quality of life and may provoke a stressful response in relatives and close friends.[3]

Treatment which aims to restore and enhance quality of life has in the past tended to be heavily dependent upon psychotropic drug therapy. Rational prescribing of anxiolytic and anti-depressant drugs will undoubtedly continue to exert considerable clinical influence. However, there is a valid case to argue that undesirable side-effects such as dependency arising out of long-term prescribing of the benzodiazepines and drowsiness or disorientation, resulting especially from the prescribing of narcoleptic drugs, may well impede rather than facilitate the development of supportive bonds with hospitals' staff, family and friends. This latter need assumes considerable status in the management of patients, where aggressive treatment of their physical disease is clearly indicated for cure.[4]

In such a situation as this, psychologic dysfunction can assume crisis proportions to a point where continued administration of potentially beneficial treatment may be threatened. Of no lesser consequence is management of those for whom cure or even palliation of disease is no longer appropriate and with whom ease and spontaneity in communication is so vitally important.

The value of behavioural intervention for the treatment of psychological dysfunction in cancer patients is becoming increasingly well documented.[5] The purpose of this paper is to follow up and to expand upon a preliminary report of the early data[6] of a study which has attempted to evaluate the role for and status of Relaxation Training (ReT), applied by a clinical psychologist, working within a hospital oncology unit. The focus of the study concentrated upon patients whose response to treatment with anxiolytic and/or anti-depressant drugs—initially prescribed by patients' own G.P.s or by hospital physicians—had had a disappointing outcome. Its successful application to compliant patients has led to its integration as part of the provision of normal supportive care available within the unit.

PATIENTS AND METHOD

Over a two-and-a-half-year period, 119 patients (approximately 15% of the total annual patient turnover) developed symptoms of chronic psychological distress. All had previously received at least one month's continuous treatment with anxiolytic or anti-depressant drugs or both, without evident improvement. Patients were referred to the department's clinical psychologist following ward rounds, or during case discussions which took place daily within the unit.

Depression was confirmed in diagnosis where patients clearly manifested evidence of depressed mood, of impairment in ability to concentrate, irritability, sadness and weepiness. Other symptoms which are also aetiologically associated with clinical depression, e.g. feelings of guilt, self-devaluation (which in cancer patients is frequently associated with self-perceived change in body-image), ideational suicide were also noted. Symptoms which, in varying degrees of intensity, are commonly associated with neurotic depression and with major depression, but which frequently are inseparable from the disease process and the effects of anti-cancer treatments, were omitted altogether, viz. loss of energy, loss of libido, sleep disturbance, loss of appetite and weight loss, etc. Chronic anxiety state was diagnosed where there was evidence of at least five of the following: loss of concentration, increased irritability, imaginative fears, fear of being alone, unaccountable bouts of nervous tension, feeling of nervous exhaustion, inappropriate panic reactions, tendency for obsessive and/or compulsive thoughts or behaviour to predominate. Biological symptoms frequently associated with acute anxiety, i.e. over-stimulation of the ANS in the form of respiratory increase, dyspnoea, dysphagia, micturition, diarrhoea, bodily weakness, etc., were omitted, for reasons stated previously. The method of assessment—which, because of the overtly distressed state of many patients, was applied verbally—has now been developed into a self-report questionnaire which is shortly to be the subject of a further publication.

Depression or anxiety state was diagnosed as being present in all 119 patients. No reliable data are available which would facilitate comparison between symptoms apparent at the time of original prescription of anxiolytic or anti-depressant drugs and those present at the time of attempted recruitment for ReT.

Of the 119 patients referred, 68 (27 males and 41 females) agreed to participate in ReT. Forty-four patients (17 males and 27 females) declined and seven patients were considered to be unsuitable because of the effects of their disease upon cognitive functioning. The principal ground for non-compliance was patients' perceived unorthodoxy of ReT. Of the 68 compliant patients, 44 (65%) and 9 (13%) were receiving chemotherapy or radiotherapy respectively.

Nine female patients (13%) were receiving hormone therapy, whilst the remaining 6 patients (9%) were off treatment altogether. Twenty-one patients (31%) were declared to be in complete or partial remission, 40 patients (59%) were progressing and the remaining 7 patients had stable disease. Chi square analysis was carried out, comparing males and females on the variables of "nature of treatment being received" and "ECOG status" statistical comparability was clearly indicated.

Relaxation training, as it was introduced and applied in actual therapy sessions, entailed three distinct yet interrelated stages:

1. A credible and acceptable rationale as the basis for the development of ReT as a precise coping skill.
2. Actual training in ReT.
3. A feasible and acceptable strategy for its self-administration.

These sequential stages may be summarized in the following manner:

An informal analysis and, where necessary, modification of the patient's present and future time perception was attempted. Patients were asked to rank their present needs in order of self-perceived importance. They were also encouraged to assess and to compare levels of ability to cope with their present circumstances. A rationale for the application of profound relaxation as a potential means of mobilizing an inherent resource was also provided. Relaxation training initially involved the application of simple breathing exercises, aided by visualization of relaxing imagery, e.g. the ebb and flow of waves on the sea shore, etc. A modified version of the original Jacobson technique for progressive muscle relaxation (PMR)[7, 8] was introduced and applied in accordance with a precise format, in which patients were encouraged to relax one gross-muscle group at a time by the "tense–relax" method. Attention was repeatedly focused upon the somatic component of tension and of relaxation being experienced in particular muscle groups. Such relaxation was further facilitated by means of a lightly-induced hypnosis employing the well-documented "ego-strengthening" routine,[9] adapted to encompass the individual patient's psychologic needs and goals.

Training sessions in ReT were undertaken individually with hospitalized patients, or with outpatients attending the treatment unit. Each ReT therapy session took approximately 30 minutes to complete and a further identical session took place on each of the first two days.

Patients were encouraged to report any beneficial and adverse effects experienced. The requirement for continued application and training was met by means of a self-administered audio tape-recording of the actual therapy session. Headphones were routinely employed in an attempt to simulate the original experience as well as to eliminate competing auditory stimuli. Two such tape-recorded sessions were staged on the third day and thereafter, until self-administration of ReT was satisfactorily achieved.

Compliant patients were interviewed again, by the one of us (SB) who had carried out the patient assessment described earlier. These further interviews took place at intervals of 48 hours, 1 week, 2 weeks and 1 month after the commencement of ReT. However, it is appreciated that in the absence (for reasons stated previously) of psychometric data, results based upon the outcome of such interviews, carried out by the member of staff who was also involved in the administration of ReT, would possess little or no reportable value. It was therefore decided to employ an alternative method for assessment of the experienced and observed effects of ReT. Such assessments were in fact carried out by the patients themselves, by close relatives and by senior members of nursing and of medical staff. This ensured that any reference to change, or its absence, would be based upon four independent ratings. Moreover, it followed that such ratings could be confirmed, or otherwise, by reference to computation of the level of consensus achieved. A single page questionnaire was devised to standardize this process. Considerable emphasis was placed upon:

1. The experimental nature of ReT for cancer patients with its attendant need, eventually to evaluate its usefulness in a randomized trial.
2. The ensuing need for absolute honesty and impartiality in response.

Responses of the four groups of raters were elicited at intervals of 48 hours, 1 week and 1 month and were related to three criteria for assessment, viz. "psychologic", "social" and "other behavioural".

"Psychologic" change was confined to observed/reported ability to exert self-control over thoughts and feelings and to remain calm and controlled for extended periods. Change in "social" functioning was indicated by observed/reported recovery of ability to satisfactorily inter-relate with relatives, with members of medical and nursing staff and with other patients to normal levels. "Other behavioural" change was indicated by observed/reported change in the onset, duration and overall quality of night sleep.

Assessment of results achieved were made in accordance with the following categories:

0 = No change
1 = Some improvement
2 = Return to normal functioning

Within such a context as this, normal behaviour is notoriously difficult to define. It is used here to denote the level of performance acknowledged and regarded by individual patients and other raters as being that which approximated to normality on the basis of prior knowledge of the person concerned.

The index of agreement, "kappa" (K),[10] has been developed in order to accurately assess scales of diagnostic category. Its further refinement, "weighted kappa" (Kw), provides an appropriately weighted index of such diagnostic category where 0 = chance agreement and 1 = perfect agreement. This method for statistical evaluation of the level of concordance which is apparent in reported results was chosen as being the most appropriate method of analysis.

RESULTS

Of the 27 males who originally participated in the study, six did not continue through to completion. Five patients were lost to the study by death and one by default, due to lack of interest. One male participant reported "no change" throughout the entire period of his participation in the study.

Of the 41 female participants, there was unanimous agreement concerning two patients who failed to report or to show evidence of improvement (the first discontinued during the first week and the second died toward the end of the second week). A further two female patients manifested continued social withdrawal although reporting and manifesting "psychologic" and "other behavioural" improvement. In all, eight female patients were lost to the study, five by death and three by default.

With the exception of nine patients (seven males, two females) who were not subject to assessment by nursing staff, all participants in the study were subject to the process of assessment as described previously. All nine such exceptions were in fact seen as outpatients at a different hospital location which employs different nursing personnel to those regular members of oncology nursing staff engaged exclusively within the treatment unit.

The calculated Kw of 0.85 (males) and 0.9 (females) for results shown in Table 1 indicates a high level of concordance between the four classes of raters.

TABLE 1. ASSESSMENT OF PATIENTS' RESPONSE

		Males (n 27)									Females (n 41)								
		48 hrs			1 week			1 month*			48 hrs			1 week*			1 month*		
		0	1	2	0	1	2	0	1	2	0	1	2	0	1	2	0	1	2
Psychologic	Patients	4	7	16	4	7	16	3	6	12	3	9	29	2	9	28	—	6	27
	Relatives	4	5	18	3	7	17	3	6	12	2	10	29	1	9	29	—	4	29
	Medical	4	8	15	4	8	15	3	8	10	4	10	27	3	9	27	—	9	24
	Nursing**	2	5	13	2	5	13	1	5	8	3	8	28	3	8	26	—	6	25
Social	Patients	4	7	16	5	6	16	3	6	12	3	10	28	2	9	28	2	4	27
	Relatives	4	5	18	4	7	16	3	6	12	2	11	28	1	9	29	0	4	29
	Medical	4	8	15	5	8	14	3	8	10	4	11	26	3	11	25	3	6	24
	Nursing**	2	5	13	2	5	13	1	5	8	3	10	26	3	10	24	3	5	23
Other	Patients	1	7	19	1	6	20	2	5	14	3	9	29	2	9	28	—	5	28
Behavioural	Relatives	1	8	18	—	7	20	2	5	14	3	10	28	2	9	28	—	5	28
	Medical	2	6	19	1	6	20	2	5	14	3	9	29	2	11	26	—	5	28
	Nursing**	—	4	16	—	3	17	—	3	11	3	8	28	2	10	25	—	4	27

* Numbers reduced by death or default, i.e. six males and eight females.

** Some subjects were not assessed by nursing staff (see text).

0 = no change; 1 = some improvement; 2 = return to normal functioning.

DISCUSSION

Reactive ability training has been shown to be suitable for patients suffering from other stress-inducing physical illnesses.[11-13] Our interest was in its applied value to the cancer patient.

Due emphasis should be placed upon the fact that this study is but the first of a series of studies on the use and the value of ReT which are currently being undertaken in this department. One major contribution of this particular study therefore resides in its capacity to inform about the need for consequent modification and refinement.

Since it is obviously the case that the method of assessment is so vitally important to the reporting of results, it is necessary to discuss and to comment upon the method which was employed in this study. Without doubt, an appropriate form of psychometric evaluation—preferably, of course, employing a validated scale for the measurement of anxiety and/or depression—would have been our first choice. In the event, this was simply not possible for a considerable number of patients. Quite apart from the level of indisposition being experienced by many patients—sufficient to deter their completion of a self-report type questionnaire—such an attempt to so engage them made at this time would have been suspect ethically and almost certainly would have lost the co-operation and goodwill of near relatives. In this clinical situation, sensitivity and sound practice for eliciting genuine responses was our aim.

The method which, in the event, was adopted and which has been described previously, was selected for a number of reasons. Firstly, it involved patients and their close relatives. Information obtained from these sources is of consummate importance and so long as care is taken to adequately brief such persons concerning the utter futility of incorrect or even exaggerated responses, there is little likelihood of faking. Second, the deployment of a single-sheet questionnaire facilitated an element of standardization to the responses which were being elicited from the various sources. Thirdly, it provided data which could thereafter be analysed so as to determine statistically, the level of concordance achieved.

The major benefits which appear to be associated with ReT and which have been reported by patients and other raters may be summarized as follows:

1. Rapid overall improvement in psychologic state with immediate enhancement of quality of life.

2. Improvement in onset and duration of night sleep.
3. Easier medical supervision and nursing care.
4. Improvement in psychological tolerance of anti-cancer treatments.
5. More appropriate management in terminal care.
6. Minimal requirement for psychotropic drugs.
7. Reduced requirement for analgesia.

It was only to be expected that departure from conventional and well-known therapies would produce a substantial number of refusals. Compliance was slightly higher among males than among females, although males showed greater reluctance toward continued self-management of ReT once improvement had been achieved. Compliant patients who were also in the terminal stages of their illnesses appeared to obtain help and support from ReT right up to the time of death. The overall sustained benefit experienced and reported by patients has led to the adoption of ReT as a routinely available supportive treatment within this unit. In selected cases it has taken precedence over the use of psychotropic drugs for the management of psychologic dysfunction, although rational prescribing of anxiolytic and anti-depressant drugs will undoubtedly continue to possess unique significance and value.

A further principal advantage of ReT resides in its apparent capacity to mobilize a resource for self-control which is essentially the patient's own. This is especially valuable in a chemotherapy unit where the busy technologic atmosphere might be conducive to the reinforcement of feelings of passivity among patients. Moreover, it appears to reduce the sense of loneliness and isolation which some patients are known to feel and which may actually be exacerbated by the administration of certain mood-modifying and pain-relieving drugs.

No formal record—for the purpose of research and future reporting—was kept concerning the forty-four subjects who declined ReT. However, on the basis of ongoing clinical reports, indicating psychologic performance of members of the non-compliant group who survived for a period in excess of one month (n 35), it is clear that members of this group appeared to do far less well throughout the stated period and beyond.

It is of course entirely conceivable that ReT exerted only minimal influence in achieving such an apparently favourable response. Participant-patients were presumably committed to a belief in the possibility of improvement, as is clear from their actual compliance. Moreover, such a belief appears to have been manifestly sufficient

S. Bindemann et al

to overcome whatever inhibitions such relatively unconventional procedures may have provoked. Thus ReT may be said merely to have focused upon and to have facilitated motivation in the direction of a desire for improvement.

No attempt was made in this particular study to evaluate the unique contributions of such well-known procedures as counselling, PMR and hypnosis. The disproportionate amount of time spent in preparatory counselling, as distinct from, or in conjunction with time taken in training in PMR and hypnosis does therefore require evaluation.

Although the point concerning difficulties in designing randomized studies of treatment-procedures in which motivation is of the essence[14] is well taken, it is clear that a controlled trial would greatly enhance an objective evaluation. Such a randomized study has recently been carried out within this treatment unit.[15] Questions raised by phenomena of compliance–non-compliance have also been investigated.

It is also perfectly possible that response may be in part, a function of the individual therapist. The administration of ReT is undeniably time-consuming and there is a need to investigate whether other medical or nursing staff can readily become proficient in its administration in a modified and economical form. If this is shown to be the case, then there is no reason why ReT should not be made more routinely available to patients who are being treated for malignant as well as other serious illnesses.

The understandable fascination with quality of life, which is currently reflected in the literature concerning the treatment of malignant illness, demands more than its mere definition and evaluation as a concept. There is urgent need for studies which actively embody the pursuit of valid means to its enhancement, as a variable which shares at least an equal status with the aim for survival.

Acknowledgement.—This research was supported by a Cancer Research Campaign Grant No. CRC/XC1041/E4/2E40.

REFERENCES

1. Harris, J. G. (1978) Nausea, vomiting and cancer treatment, *CA: A Cancer Journal for Clinicians,* **28,** 194–201.
2. Holland, J. (1977) Psychological aspects of oncology. *Medical Clinics of North America,* **61,** 737–748.
3. Wellisch, D. K., Jamison, K. R. and Pasnau, R. O. (1978) Psychosocial aspects of mastectomy: the man's perspective. *American Journal of Psychiatry,* **135,** 543–546.

4. Glaus, A. (1983) Curative tumour therapy and preservation of quality of life. *Deutscher Berufsverband für Krankenpflege (Gern)*, **12**, 22–23.
5. Burish, T. G., Shartner, C. D. and Lyles, J. N. (1981) Effectiveness of multiple-site EMG biofeedback and relaxation training in reducing the aversiveness of cancer chemotherapy. *Biofeedback and Self-Regulation*, **6**, 523–535.
6. Bindemann, S., Calman, K. C., Milsted, R. A. V. and Trotter, J. M. (1981) Management of psychological stress in cancer patients, an alternative approach. *British Journal of Cancer*, **44**, 2, 291.
7. Jacobson, E. (1938) *Progressive Relaxation.* University of Chicago Press, Chicago.
8. Bernstein, D. A. and Borkøvec, T. D. (1973) *Progressive Relaxation Training: A Manual for the Helping Professions.* Research Press: Champaign, Illustrated.
9. Harland J. (1971) *Medical and Dental Hypnosis and its Clinical Application.* Bailliere-Tindall.
10. Cohen, J. (1969) Weighted kappa: nominal scales agreement with provision for scaled disagreement or partial credit. *Psychological Bulletin*, **70**, 213–220.
11. Achterberg, J., McGraw, P. and Lawlis, G. F. (1981) Rheumatoid arthritis: a study of relaxation and temperature biofeedback training as an adjunctive therapy. *Biofeedback and Self-Regulation*, **6**, 207–223.
12. Agras, W. S., Horne, M. and Taylor, C. B. (1982) Expectation and blood-pressure lowering effects of relaxation. *Psychosomatic Medicine*, **44**, 389–395.
13. Erskine-Milliss, J. and Schonell, M. (1981) Relaxation therapy in asthma: a critical review. *Psychosomatic Medicine*, **4**, 365–372.
14. Stoll, B. A. (1979) Is hope a factor in survival? In *Mind and Cancer Prognosis*, pp. 191–197 (ed. Stoll). John Wiley & Sons, Chichester.
15. Bindemann, S., Kaye, S. B., Welsh, J., Habeshaw, T. and Calman, K. C. (1986) Coping with cancer: a randomized study of relaxation training (ReT) in patient care and management. *British Journal of Cancer* (in press).

Hypnotic Techniques in the Reduction of Pain During Procedures with Paediatric Cancer Patients

R. G. LANSDOWN

ABSTRACT

It is well established that children frequently find the treatment they receive for cancer and related illnesses worse than the possible outcome. In recent years behavioural paediatricians and psychologists have turned their attention to seeking ways of helping children cope with the pain experienced during lumbar punctures and bone marrows. Controlled studies have suggested that hypnotic techniques have a place in such work, although it is clear from published work that not all children are likely to respond.

As with all forms of behavioural treatment, a detailed behavioural analysis must be made before any intervention is attempted. Part of this analysis includes subjective ratings of pain along with observers' ratings. Pain measurement is not without its pitfalls and these are discussed.

The results of studies carried out in America are presented, along with an outline of research that is currently being planned by the author.

The Effectiveness of Specialist Nurses as Oncology Counsellors

M. WATSON

ABSTRACT

Studies where nurses have provided counselling for cancer patients are briefly reviewed. The nurse-counsellor service for breast cancer patients at King's College Hospital, London, is described and some results are presented from an evaluation of this service. As a result of counselling, patients appear to make a more rapid adjustment following treatment by mastectomy and enhanced feelings of control. It was concluded that the results from this evaluation are encouraging, but more evidence is needed before recommending that this service should be made more widely available.

In 1979 a specialist nurse was appointed to the Department of Surgery at King's College Hospital, London,* to provide a counselling service for women with breast cancer. This service was subsequently evaluated in a controlled prospective trial and some results for this evaluation are presented.

There are many reasons for evaluating supportive therapy. At present the evidence relating to the benefits patients derive is somewhat equivocal.[1] A brief overview of some recent studies,[2-7] where support was offered by among others specialist nurses, indicates that no clear trends have emerged (Table 1).

If any trend can be observed, it is simply that individual counselling appears to be slightly more effective overall than group counselling. In addition, studies examining the rates of psychological morbidity among patients with early breast cancer[8,9] have indicated that approximately 70–75% do not suffer any severe disturbance in affect (that is, profound enough to merit labelling as a

* This nurse is generously supported by the Cancer Research Campaign.

17

psychiatric "case"). Therefore, the provision of counselling services needs to be justified on two counts: that a significant need exists and that benefits will be derived from this type of support.

Before describing the evaluation of the counselling service offered at King's College Hospital, it might be useful to say something about its nature.

TABLE 1. REVIEW OF SUPPORT STUDIES

Ferlic *et al.*	↑ Confidence in medical staff
Golonka	Anxiety—no difference
Spiegel *et al.*	↓ Mood disturbance
	Self-esteem ⎫
	Denial ⎬ no difference
	Health locus on control ⎭
Gordon *et al.*	↓ Post discharge negative affect
Linn *et al.*	↓ Depression
	↑ Life satisfaction
	↑ Internal control
	↑ Self-esteem
Maguire *et al.*	↑ Post-operative (at 4 months) anxiety

An individual counselling service was offered to all new breast cancer patients immediately the diagnosis was known. The counsellor was present when the diagnosis was given and talked to patients afterwards. Where possible, she saw patients at home before admission and then again after admission and before surgery. The counsellor then saw patients on at least one occasion post-operatively prior to discharge from hospital. This was followed by a home visit approximately two to three weeks later. The service then continued on demand, with the counsellor seeing her clients at follow-up clinics and sometimes at home. If a recurrence of the cancer was diagnosed, then counselling would recommence.

Although the content of counselling was tailored to individual needs, a general framework was adopted which covered three areas. These were: (1) emotional support and facilitation of coping and adjustment, (2) information about breast cancer and its treatment, (3) practical advice, particularly relating to the fitting and wearing of a prosthesis. Areas (2) and (3) are not usually considered to be counselling, but they are complementary aspects of the service offered and usually overlap.

EMOTIONAL SUPPORT AND FACILITATION OF COPING

The counsellor's first task was to establish the patient's priorities; that is, she ascertained what were the focal worries. They would then discuss these worries together and the patient was encouraged to express feelings. In this way she was provided with an opportunity to ventilate emotions. The patient was encouraged toward constructive methods of coping and feelings of control were promoted by involving the patient in decision making. She was also encouraged to draw upon her own resources when trying to adjust. Discussions were not confined to problems arising from the cancer diagnosis and treatment, but other problems preventing adjustment were included. Where necessary, patients were referred to other agencies for specialist advice and psychiatric referrals were made when severe reactions occurred.

EVALUATION OF COUNSELLING

The study undertaken to evaluate counselling was set up as a prospective controlled trial.

Subjects

Patients who participated in the evaluation were all diagnosed as having an early stage breast cancer which was treated by mastectomy.

Method

New patients were allocated, on a randomized fortnightly time period basis, to receive either routine care or routine care plus counselling, and 40 patients were randomized to the two groups using this procedure. Psychosocial assessments were made on three occasions: (1) one week post-operatively, whilst still on the ward, usually on the day prior to discharge, (2) three months' post-operatively, and (3) 12 months' post-operatively. The 3- and 12-month assessments were made when the patients returned to the clinic for a physical check-up. These assessments were made by one

M. Watson

of three independent interviewers* with the rotation of interviewers occurring on a random basis. Demographic, medical and psychosocial details were obtained using medical notes and a structured interview. Psychological morbidity was measured using the Profile of Mood States.[10] At the 3- and 12-months' assessments some of these areas were covered again along with some new areas. In particular, areas of worry were covered using an especially designed checklist.** Patients also completed a health locus of control questionnaire.[11] During follow-up interviews they were also asked about their satisfaction or dissatisfaction with the prosthesis and the fitting service provided.

Results

Scores on the Profile of Mood States indicated that (Table 2) at 3 months' post-operatively the counselled patients were significantly less depressed than patients receiving routine care ($p<.05$). They also showed increased feelings of vigour over the period between 1 week to 3 months' post-operatively ($p<.01$). The overall trend in both groups was toward a decrease in depression and increase in vigour throughout the year following mastectomy, but this occurred more rapidly if patients were counselled. Thus the period of distress appeared to be reduced for patients who were counselled.

TABLE 2. MEAN SCORES FOR DEPRESSION AND VIGOUR ON THE PROFILE OF MOOD STATES

Length of post-operative assessment	1 week	3 months	12 months
Depression			
Counselled	37	33*	34
Routine Care	39	37	34**
Vigour (Ebullience)			
Counselled	57	63†	64
Routine Care	58	60	65††

* When compared with the routine care group at 3 months $p<.05$
** When compared with scores for the same group at 3 months $p<.05$
† When compared with scores for the same group at 1 week $p<.01$
†† When compared with scores for the same group at 1 week $p<.05$
(All 2-tailed tests)

* S. Blake, M. Buckley and M. Watson.
** Details are available from the author.

There were also differences in health-related beliefs when these were assessed using a health locus of control scale (Table 3). Comparisons indicated that counselled patients were significantly more likely to report greater internal (i.e. personal) control when this was assessed at 3 months (p<.03). At 12 months' post-operatively they were still more likely to report greater feelings of internal control than the routine care group, but the difference was no longer statistically significant.

TABLE 3. MEAN SCORES FOR HEALTH LOCUS OF CONTROL

Length of post-operative assessment	3 months	12 months
Internal (Personal) Control		
Counselled	28*	26
Routine Care	22	23

* When compared with the routine care group at 3 months p<.03 (2-tailed test).

Four areas of reported problems were assessed (Table 4) using an especially designed questionnaire. Although there were no significant differences between the groups, patients who were counselled showed a tendency toward reporting fewer problems in all areas at the 3 months' assessment. At 12 months' post-operatively the groups were similar in their reporting of problems experienced.

TABLE 4. MEAN SCORES FOR REPORTED PROBLEMS

	Counselled group	Routine care group
At 3 months		
Body image	3.8	4.4
Sexual	3.1	3.6
Health related	4.0	5.1
Dependency	3.5	3.9
At 12 months		
Body image	3.2	3.3
Sexual	3.1	3.1
Health related	4.1	4.5
Dependency	3.5	3.6

N.B. The maximum score obtainable was 12, with high scores indicating more problems.

Data on the demand for counselling indicated just how high was the level of use of this service. All counselled patients were seen on at least four of five occasions during the pre- and immediate post-operative period. Following this, counselling was available if requested by the patient. All patients in the counselled group asked for further counselling session. The mean number of sessions requested was six, making an average of four to eleven sessions in total. Most of these subsequent sessions were devoted to counselling rather than prosthetic advice. There was, however, a great deal of variability in demand, with the range of additional sessions requested, over the year following mastectomy, extending from two to fifteen. Although this highlighted the variability in need for counselling, on average the demand was quite high.

CONCLUSIONS

A number of conclusions were drawn from this evaluation of counselling. In relation to mood state, it would appear that both groups of patients continued to adjust during the year following mastectomy, but this occurred more rapidly if they were counselled. Beliefs in internal (personal) control over health were enhanced as a result of counselling. The importance of these feelings of personal effectiveness and control for successful adjustment has been highlighted in a study by Bloom.[12] In this counselling service, patients were encouraged to draw upon their own resources in order to cope. Information was also provided to help reduce misconceptions about cancer and the uncertainties associated with the side- and after-effects of treatment. These factors may have contributed to the greater feeling of personal control reported by counselled patients. A trend was observed toward fewer problems being reported among the counselled group, although this was not statistically significant. Finally, the demand for counselling was quite high despite a wide variability in the number of sessions requested.

There are, however, a number of unresolved issues. For instance, it is important to learn which aspects of counselling are most beneficial and more feedback is needed on this from patients. Also, more data are needed to confirm the trends observed in this study. Finally, it could be argued that the effectiveness of this service was due to the idiosyncratic qualities of this counsellor. Further studies are needed to confirm that the benefits arose as a result of this type of service rather than this nurse's individual qualities.

The results from this study are encouraging, but more evidence is needed before it is possible to recommend that this support method should be more widely available.

REFERENCES

1. Watson, M. (1983) Psychosocial intervention with cancer patients: a review. *Psychological Medicine,* **13,** 839–846.
2. Ferlic, M., Goldman, A. and Kennedy, B. J. (1979) Group counselling in adult patients with advanced cancer. *Cancer,* **43,** 760–766.
3. Golonka, L. M. (1977) The use of group counselling with breast cancer patients receiving chemotherapy. *Dissertation Abstracts International,* **37**(10–A), 6362–6363.
4. Spiegel, D. and Yalom, I. D. (1978) A support group for dying patients. *International Journal of Group Psychotherapy,* **28,** 233–245.
5. Gordon, W. A., Freidenbergs, I., Diller, L., Hibberd, M., Wolf, C., Levine, L., Lipkins, R., Ezrachi, O. and Lucido, D. (1980) Efficacy of psychosocial intervention with cancer patients. *Journal of Consulting and Clinical Psychology,* **48**(6), 743–759.
6. Linn, M. W., Linn, B. S. and Harris, R. (1982) Effects of counselling for late stage cancer patients. *Cancer,* **49**(5), 1048–1055.
7. Maguire, G. P., Tait, A., Brooke, M., Thomas, C. and Sellwood, R. (1980) The effects of monitoring on the psychiatric morbidity associated with mastectomy. *British Medical Journal,* **ii,** 1454.
8. Morris, T., Greer, S. and White, P. (1977) Psychological and social adjustment to mastectomy: a two-year follow-up study. *Cancer,* **40,** 2381–2387.
9. Maguire, G. P., Lee, E. G., Bevington, D. J., Kuchemann, C. J., Crabtree, R. J. and Cornell, C. E. (1978) Psychiatric problems in the first year after mastectomy. *British Medical Journal,* **i,** 963–965.
10. McNair, D., Lorr, M. and Dropplemann, L. *Manual for Profile of Mood States.* San Diego, CA, Educational and Industrial Testing Service, 1971.
11. Wallston, K. A. and Wallston, B. S. (1982) Who is responsible for your health: The construct of health locus of control. In: *Social Psychology of Health and Illness.* Eds. Sanders, G., Suls, J. and Hillsdale, N. J. Erlbaum & Associates.
12. Bloom, J. R. (1979) Psychosocial measurement and specific hypotheses: A research note. *Journal of Consulting and Clinical Psychology,* **47,** 637–639.

SECTION TWO

Issues in Psycho-Oncology

The Assessment of Symptoms and Mood in Terminally Ill Cancer Patients

B. J. LUNT

ABSTRACT

One of the principal goals of the care of advanced cancer patients is the relief of physical and emotional distress.

The assessment of symptoms and mood states is therefore essential in evaluating the care of terminally ill cancer patients, and also in studying the effectiveness of palliative treatment. A variety of methods have been used in the past for making such assessments.

In different studies, visual analogue scales (VASs), numerical and categorical scales, and multiple item questionnaires and inventories have been completed by patients, their relatives, and by nursing and medical staff. Often the validity and reliability of these methods has not been demonstrated. Furthermore, all methods suffer from the problem of under-reporting of the severity and duration of distress. Partly this arises from a common reluctance to acknowledge distress even when asked. However, with very ill people the effects of lost data may be a more significant cause of bias, since more data are lost when people are feeling particularly ill.

Pain, nausea, breathlessness, mood and anxiety were assessed in a comparative study of hospice and hospital care for terminally ill cancer patients. Regular assessments were made, three times a week, throughout the patients' stay in the hospice or hospital. Five-point scales were used by the researcher to record the responses of the patient to direct questioning about these symptoms and mood states. The patient then completed VASs for the same symptoms and mood states.

Results relate to the reliability and validity of the interviewer-completed five-point scales, and the degree of under-reporting which arises from the use of patient completed VASs compared with interviewer-completed five-point scales.

The Surgeon's Dilemmas in the Management of the Patient with Breast Cancer

C. RAY

ABSTRACT

The surgeon is said to play a key role in helping the patient to adjust to her breast cancer, yet patients' emotions and concerns are often inadequately dealt with in the context of routine care. A study of surgeons' perceptions of breast cancer and mastectomy, and of their relationship with patients, yielded data relevant to three main areas of uncertainty and conflict which can influence the degree and nature of the support that they offer. These related to difficulties in:

(1) controlling the disease.
(2) deciding what to tell patients.
(3) talking with patients about their feelings.

In making these issues explicit, surgeons may be in a better position to cope with the ambiguities of their role and to determine its scope and limitations. They are issues that should also be explored in training, and most of the surgeons in our sample said that they would welcome more discussion of this nature at that time.

There are a number of ways in which the patient with breast cancer might be given psychological support. Group therapy, mastectomy volunteers, early intervention by psychologists or psychiatrists, counselling by specialist nurses, might all help to prevent problems from arising or reduce distress, but these facilities are not widely available. In practice most patients will have to rely upon the doctors and nurses responsible for their routine care for any support beyond that which they can obtain from family and friends. The surgeon in particular has been cited as having a key or pivotal role in determining a patient's adjustment to early breast cancer,[1, 2] and

29

Shelp[3] has argued that the doctor's "sustaining presence" can ideally provide a context not just in which a patient comes to cope with illness, but also learns the nature of the human condition and develops the character necessary to negotiate reality. In practice, however, patients complain that their psychological needs are not fully addressed in the surgeon-patient relationship. Lee and Maguire[4] have noted that signs of distress are often unnoticed or are ignored in outpatients' clinics and even cases of emotional disturbance that require specialist help remain undetected.[5, 6] The surgeon's task is a difficult one at many levels, and there are a number of conflicts and uncertainties inherent in his role which can affect the degree and nature of the support he offers. These are the subject of this paper. The data cited were obtained from a project which explored surgeons' perceptions of (a) breast cancer and mastectomy, (b) the doctor-patient relationship in this context. Twenty surgeons took part in two interviews, which explored in some depth the issues and viewpoints salient in the group, and then a questionnaire was constructed to reflect the themes emphasized by them in interview. It was sent to 42 surgeons, comprising all of those at registrar level and above with experience of breast cancer patients, at three teaching and one local hospital in the U.K. Thirty-six of the questionnaires were returned, and this pleasing degree of co-operation goes some way to offset the smallness of the sample. It has to be acknowledged that the sample are not likely to be representative of surgeons in the U.K., and that the data are most meaningful if they are regarded as reflecting the *range* of issues and viewpoints which concern surgeons, rather than too much weight being attached to the actual numbers espousing particular viewpoints. This paper will focus upon three areas of uncertainty in handling the breast cancer patient that the surgeons described, uncertainties which are inherent in their own role and which have a bearing upon the doctor-patient relationship. More detailed reports can be found in other publications.[7-9]

CONTROLLING THE DISEASE

The outcome of breast cancer is always unpredictable in the individual case, and many surgeons feel frustrated by both lack of understanding of the disease and the ineffectiveness of treatment. On the questionnaire, seven said that their primary feeling in this situation was one of frustration, seven said they mainly felt a sense of challenge, while 17 said that they experienced both equally. Many had doubts about mastectomy as a procedure, not only on grounds of its unreliability as a cure but also because of its distastefulness. Ten said they derived the same satisfaction from doing this compared with other operations, six said somewhat less, and 18 said they derived much less satisfaction. When they were asked to compare a modified radical with simple mastectomy, and simple mastectomy with local wide excision, for their effects on quantity of life and quality of life respectively, a mirror image pattern emerged—those procedures regarded as having the most positive impact on extending life were seen as having the most negative impact on its quality. There are thus conflicting criteria for determining which treatment to choose. Moreover, even in terms of survival alone, some surgeons are less than fully confident that they make the right decisions. Only two said that they were very confident, 22 that they were fairly confident, and 12 that they were not confident. When we consider how the surgeon can help the patient cope with her uncertainties and the emotional conflicts associated with the illness and its treatment, it is well to remember that he too has his own uncertainties and conflicts to deal with, even at the level of the technical aspects of his role.

INFORMING THE PATIENT

An issue which will more directly affect the surgeon's relationship with the patient is that of what she should be told about her illness. The giving of information might seem to be a way of supporting the patient and catering for her needs, but some surgeons felt that the patient can best be supported and her needs best met if information is withheld. Twenty said on the questionnaire that they tended toward openness, six that they tended towards discretion, while nine said that for them the two were evenly balanced. To be more specific, they were asked to say with what percentage of patients they employed five different strategies which had commonly been described in the interview. At the extremes, surgeons said that they would openly and frankly discuss cancer with 18% of patients, and reassure the patient that it is not cancer or avoid discussing the illness with only 3%. For the majority of patients, the preferred strategies were to discuss cancer but with a bias toward reassurance in presenting the facts (53%), or to discuss the illness and its implications but avoiding the terms

C. Ray

"cancer" or "malignancy" (27%). As a group the surgeons believed that the vast majority of patients are definitely aware of their cancer by the time of mastectomy (84%) or have some awareness (12%).

TALKING ABOUT FEELINGS

To provide adequately for patients' psychological needs, the surgeon should, however, do more than offer the information he feels appropriate. He should also be alert to her worries and concerns. Only seven of the surgeons said on the questionnaire that they asked directly about feelings; the others said that they would do so only if the patient raised the issue herself or was showing obvious signs of concern. Few thought that they had a good knowledge of a patient's reaction either to her cancer or to the loss of the breast: six and five respectively. This is in part a question of role definition. A minority thought talking with the patient about her feelings to be a key aspect of their role. They defined this role, primarily, in terms of making decisions about diagnosis and treatment and conveying confidence in these areas, and, secondarily, in terms of providing information and general reassurance (Table 1). There are, however, other barriers. One is the fear that, in entering into a discussion of the patients' emotions, the surgeon might place his professional detachment in jeopardy. Another is that many surgeons feel they lack the skills that would be necessary for this kind of relationship. Twelve said that they felt "rather uncertain" when talking about the patient's feelings with her, and only one said that he felt "very confident". They expressed slightly less confidence in this respect than in deciding what information to give the patient about her illness (Table 2).

TABLE 1. ASPECT OF THE SURGEON'S ROLE: NO. OF SURGEONS VIEWING THESE AS OF KEY IMPORTANCE

making the right diagnosis	36
deciding on treatment	33
conveying competence	26
informing about treatment	20
giving overt reassurance	19
informing about the illness	15
discussing feelings about the illness	12
discussing feelings about mastectomy	7

TABLE 2. CONFIDENCE IN GIVING INFORMATION AND DISCUSSING THE PATIENT'S FEELINGS (NO. OF SURGEONS).

	Deciding what to tell	Talking about feelings
Very uncertain	0	0
Rather uncertain	4	12
Fairly confident	26	23
Very confident	6	1

In conclusion, surgeons are subjected to uncertainty and stress as part of their role both in managing the disease and in managing their relationship with patients. There are ambiguities about the understanding of cancer, about the relative merits of treatment alternatives and about the criteria to be used in assessing these. Then, in addition, they have to decide what information to offer and how to present it, trying to meet the patient's desire for certainty in an uncertain situation, and her desire for reassurance where reassurance might be inappropriate, and trying to achieve a balance between dispelling ignorance, on the one hand, and not dispelling hope on the other. Finally, they have to consider to what extent it is their responsibility to address themselves to patients' needs for emotional support and to what extent they have the skills to do this. In our study, surgeons articulated these conflicts and in so doing we would hope that they and their colleagues might be better placed to recognize and to resolve them. These are also the kinds of issues that could usefully be explored in training, and the majority of our sample said that they would welcome more discussion of what to tell patients and how to talk with them about their feelings at that time. Some studies have shown that opportunities to interview or listen to patients, and seminars and discussion groups can help to modify students' perceptions of the cancer experience[10] and to increase their empathy.[11] It may be that such training would be most fruitful at a later stage, when the surgeon is in role and has had some direct experience of the issues. The following could then be more specifically addressed: how to assess the patient's need for information, how to monitor her reactions effectively, and how to fulfil the general ideal of the "sustaining presence" that Shelp[3] has elaborated.

REFERENCES

1. Ervin, C. J. (1973) Psychological adjustment to mastectomy. *Medical Aspects of Human Sexuality*, **7**, 42–65.
2. Klein, R. (1971) A crisis on grow on. *Cancer*, **28**, 1660–1665.
3. Shelp, E. E. (1984) Courage: a neglected virtue in the patient-physician relationship. *Social Science and Medicine*, **18**, 351–360.
4. Lee, E. C. G. and Maguire, G. P. (1975) Emotional distress in patients attending a breast clinic. *British Journal of Surgery*, **62**, 162.
5. Maguire, G. P. (1976) The psychological and social sequelae of mastectomy. In *Modern Perspectives in the Psychiatric Aspects of Surgery* (J. G. Howells, ed.), pp. 390–421. Brunner/Mazel, New York.
6. Maguire, P., Tait, A., Brooke, M., Thomas, C. and Sellwood, R. (1980) Effect of counselling on the psychiatric morbidity associated with mastectomy. *British Medical Journal*, **2**, 1454–1456.
7. Ray, C., Fisher, J. and Lindop, J. (1984) The surgeon-patient relationship in the context of breast cancer. *International Review of Applied Psychology*, **33**, 531–543.
8. Ray, C. and Baum, M. (1985) *Psychological Aspects of Early Breast Cancer*. Springer Verlag.
9. Ray, C., Fisher, J. and Wisniewski, T. K. M. (in press). Surgeons' attitudes toward breast cancer: their perceptions of the illness and its treatment, and of their role in relation to the patient. *Journal of Psychosocial Oncology*.
10. Cassileth, B. R. and Egan, T. A. (1969) Modification of medical students' perceptions of the cancer experience. *Journal of Medical Education*, **10**, 797–802.
11. Poole, A. D. and Sanson-Fisher, R. W. (1979) Understanding the patient: A neglected aspect of medical education. *Social Science and Medicine*, **13A**, 37–43.

Measurement of Psychological Morbidity in Advanced Breast Cancer

P. HOPWOOD

ABSTRACT

Although there has been extensive research into the psychosocial sequelae of treatments of early breast cancer, little attention has been paid to psychiatric disorders in patients with advanced cancer of the breast. A pilot study was conducted to determine the psychological morbidity in a group of 26 patients attending a clinic for chemotherapy. Patients were assessed using a standard psychiatric interview before commencing treatment, and 2–3 months later. Depressive illness or anxiety states requiring further intervention occurred in nine patients (35%) overall. In five (19%) illness occurred before chemotherapy, and during chemotherapy in four (15%). Depression and anxiety states responded to anxiolytic or antidepressant medication in the majority of patients.

It was concluded that at least one-third of patients presenting with advanced breast cancer may have psychological morbidity amenable to treatment. A further study was piloted to test the feasibility of monitoring patients' psychological status at each clinic visit, using a self-rating questionnaire. Such an approach was found to be both acceptable to patients and feasible to administer using clinic personnel.

There has now been extensive research into the psychosocial sequelae of early breast cancer and its treatment.[1-3] In contrast, very little attention has been focused on the plight of patients with progressive disease who have to cope with increasing loss of body integrity and function, to accept pain and discomfort from disease and/or its treatment, and try to come to terms with a fatal condition.

In addition to this obvious gap in the research literature, there has been growing concern at a clinical level to improve the quality of life for these patients.

PSYCHOLOGICAL MORBIDITY IN PATIENTS WITH ADVANCED BREAST CANCER

In Manchester, therefore, a pilot study was conducted to determine the psychological morbidity in a group of women with advanced breast cancer.[4] A series of 26 new referrals to the breast clinic of the Christie Hospital were evaluated; all these patients were to receive chemotherapy for the treatment of metastatic disease. Patients were assessed on two occasions: before commencing treatment and 2–3 months later. Interviews were carried out during a routine hospital visit and conducted by a clinical psychiatrist using a standard interview schedule.[5] These interviews were normally audiotaped to allow reliability checks to be carried out later.

A diagnosis of depressive illness or an anxiety state was made according to strict diagnostic criteria as used in routine clinical practice, and psychiatric disorder classified according to the diagnostic categories of the ICD (*International Classification of Diseases*, ninth revision, World Health Organization, 1975). On this basis, depressive illness or anxiety states occurred in nine patients (35%) overall. In five (19%) such illness occurred before commencing chemotherapy, and during chemotherapy in four (15%). A further three patients died during the study period and did not complete assessment. Reactive depression was the most frequent diagnosis, occurring in eight patients; in two of these women an anxiety state was concurrent, whereas in one patient an anxiety state was the primary diagnosis. Although these reactions were clearly understandable, they also warranted intervention, and it was noted that the majority responded to anxiolytic or anti-depressant medication prescribed as part of the routine clinical management of these patients.

It was concluded that up to one-third of patients presenting with, and being treated for, advanced breast cancer may have psychological morbidity amenable to treatment. This level of morbidity is comparable to the findings of Plumb and Holland,[6] who reported clinically significant depression in 20–30% of patients admitted for the treatment of advanced cancer.

MONITORING PSYCHOLOGICAL STATUS

It was decided, to try and screen routinely a population of patients with advanced breast cancer attending for chemotherapy in two out-patient clinics in South Manchester. A further study was piloted to test the feasibility of monitoring patients' psychological status at each clinic visit, using a self-rating questionnaire. A total of 45 patients were invited to take part in the study, of whom three (7%) declined. Twenty-four patients were evaluable at the time of analysis of the results; these patients had all completed a pre-treatment questionnaire together with a series of at least four further self-rating scales, usually at monthly intervals. Patients not evaluable had either died, failed to complete a sufficient number of questionnaires, or completed them incorrectly.

The questionnaire used was the Rotterdam Symptom Checklist for cancer patients developed by Pruyn, de Haes and their co-workers in Holland.[7, 8] This scale consists of 30 symptom items, each with four "Likert"-type responses ranging from "not at all" to "very much" and covering symptom items ranging from physical to psychological complaints. There are seven further global questions which were not analysed for the purposes of this study.

The questionnaires were found to be acceptable to patients (compliance was over 90%) on repeated usage, although one question relating to sexual activity was frequently omitted and may have been inappropriate. Self-rating scales were administered by the routine clinical personnel, usually nurses, and such an approach proved feasible even in a busy out-patient setting.

In looking at the results of this study, the questionnaire was broken down into six component subscales namely: physical complaints, psychological complaints, anxiety, depression, sexual problems and severe toxicity; only anxiety and depression will be considered here.

It was necessary to use existing threshold levels for each subscale, to indicate a possible cut-off point above which psychological morbidity was likely to exist and below which the symptom level was deemed acceptable. These threshold values had been worked out on a different population of cancer patients[9] and it was realized that although early breast cancer patients were included in that validation work, such thresholds may not be appropriate for patients with advanced disease.

Bearing in mind these limitations, the following results were found. Before commencing chemotherapy seven patients (29%) reported a significant level of anxiety symptoms (i.e. at or above the threshold value), and five patients (21%) rated themselves depressed at this time (i.e. their scores were above the threshold value on the depression subscale). During each month of the treatment period 33–42% of patients self-rated above the threshold level for anxiety symptoms, and 38–46% rated themselves depressed. Overall, up to two-thirds of patients rated themselves either anxious or depressed or both, on at least one occasion during the weeks of treatment.

The questionnaire scores obtained in this way give a measure of reported symptomatology, but do not necessarily reflect the true prevalence of psychiatric morbidity. This will depend on the accuracy of the questionnaire, that is its *validity* and *reliability*.

The most important feature of any questionnaire used as a screening instrument is its clinical validity; this is defined as the measured efficiency of the instrument in correctly identifying subjects who have been independently diagnosed by a clinical psychiatrist as being psychologically ill or well. Before being able to interpret fully the results of the screening pilot study, therefore, it was necessary to undertake further calibration work in a population of advanced breast cancer patients.

This work is currently in progress, and to date nearly 200 women have completed questionnaires. Of these, 70 have been interviewed by a clinical psychiatrist using a standard interview schedule.[10] It is necessary to interview patients with both low and high scores on the questionnaires, and such patients are selected as near as possible at random so as not to introduce bias. All interviews are conducted after the completion of the self-rating scales, but on the same occasion (a routine clinic visit) and with the interviewer "blind" to the questionnaire scores. It was decided to carry out calibration work on two questionnaires in this study since both are potentially useful as screening instruments. Patients are therefore asked to complete the 30 item symptom checklist of the Rotterdam Scale, used in earlier work, together with the Hospital Anxiety and Depression Scale (HADS).[11] The HADS is a straightforward 14 item symptom checklist designed for detecting states of depression and anxiety in patients with physical illness.

In order to work out the validity of these questionnaires the sensitivity and specificity of each instrument must be calculated.

Sensitivity is the ability of the instrument to identify "cases" (that is patients diagnosed as having a psychiatric disorder) correctly and is calculated from the following ratio:

Number of true cases
———————————————————————————
Number of true cases + False negative scores

It is represented as a percentage.

Specificity is the ability of the instrument to identify "non-cases" (that is patients without psychiatric disorder) correctly and is calculated from the following ratio:

$$\frac{\text{Number of true non-cases}}{\text{Number of true non-cases} + \text{False positive scores}}$$

It is also represented as a percentage.

Both questionnaires were designed so that depression and anxiety symptoms can be scored separately, and it is therefore possible to calculate the specificity and sensitivity of each subscale. If a questionnaire has a high sensitivity, it should identify a high proportion of patients with psychological disorder. If it is also highly specific, patients who are psychologically well will also be correctly identified by scores below the threshold value. Low sensitivity means that patients with problems may be missed, and low specificity means that patients will be needlessly interviewed who are in fact psychologically well.

A preliminary analysis of the data indicates that both questionnaires show potential for use in this field, but further work is required to establish their full clinical application. Firstly, we need to increase the patient sample of the validation study by continuing to interview both high and low scorers. Secondly, we need to evaluate the reliability of the questionnaires, that is the consistency of the rating scales in measuring morbidity on different occasions.

Recent work by the authors of the Rotterdam Scale has shown that this instrument should probably not be used to discriminate depression and anxiety as separate entities, but that it should be used to define a more global dimension of "psychosocial complaints". It will therefore be necessary to review the existing data using a revised subscale to take account of this.

It is also planned to carry out inter-rater reliability checks on the existing clinical interviews.

We hope to report results of this work on a future occasion; meanwhile, we also need to consider other self-rating scales for use in this area such as the General Health Questionnaire[10] and a self-rating scale recently developed in Glasgow.[12]

It is hoped that this kind of research will provide us with valuable instruments for use in screening for psychiatric morbidity in cancer patients.

REFERENCES

1. Maguire, G. P., Lee, E. G., Bevington, D. S., Kuchemann, C. S., Crabtree, R. J. and Cornell, C. E. (1978) Psychiatric problems in the first year after mastectomy. *British Medical Journal*, **I**, 963–965.

PIMD-D

P. Hopwood

2. Morris, T., Greer, H. S. and White, P. (1977) Psychological and social adjustment to mastectomy: a two-year follow up study. Cancer, **40**, 3281-3287.

3. Weisman, A. D. and Worden, J. W. (1977) Coping and vulnerability in cancer patients. Research report, Project Omega. Harvard Medical School, Boston, Mass., USA.

4. Hopwood, P. (1983) The psychological morbidity of advanced breast cancer. Unpublished MSc thesis, University of Manchester, England.

5. Goldberg, D. P., Cooper, B., Eastwood, M. R., Kedward, H. B. and Shepherd, M. (1970) A standardized psychiatric interview for use in community surveys. British Journal of Preventative and Social Medicine, **24**, 18-23.

6. Plumb, M. M. and Holland, J. (1981) Comparative studies of psychological function in patients with advanced cancer II. Interviewer rated current and past psychiatric symptoms. Psychosomatic Medicine, **43**, 243-254.

7. Pruyn, J. F. A., Van den Heuvel, W. J. A. and Jonkers, R. (1982) The development of a symptom checklist for cancer patients. Personal communication.

8. de Haes, J. C. J. M., Pruyn, J. F. A. and van Knippenberg, F. C. E. (1983) Klachtenlijst voor kankerpatienten. Eerste ervaringen. Nederlands Tijdschrift voor de Psychologie, **38**, 403-422.

9. Trew, M. and Maguire, P. (1982) Further comparison of two instruments for measuring quality of life in cancer patients. In Beckman, J. (Ed.), Proceedings Third Workshop EORTC Study Group in Quality of Life. Published by county hospital service of Fuhen, Dept. Clinical Psychology, Odense University Hospital, Denmark, pp. 111-127.

10. Goldberg, D. P. (1972) The Detection of Psychiatric Illness by Questionnaire. Oxford University Press, London.

11. Zigmond, A. S. and Snaith, R. P. (1983) The Hospital Anxiety and Depression Scale. Acta Psychiatrica Scandinavica, **67**, 361-370.

12. Bindemann, S. (1984) Personal communication.

Theories, Methods and Some Results on Coping with Cancer and Contact with Fellow Sufferers

J. F. A. PRUYN, H. W. VAN DEN BORNE
and P. STRINGER

ABSTRACT

Two hundred and sixteen patients with Hodgkin's disease (and non-Hodgkin's lymphoma) and 282 patients with breast cancer in 15 medical centres across The Netherlands were interviewed and filled out a variety of scales designed to assess their information-seeking and affiliation behaviour. Specifically, the primary purposes of the study were: (1) to gain insight into which types of patients do and which patients do not have contact with other patients and to determine the effects of this contact on their health, and (2) to determine the specific amounts and kinds of information needed by patients to cope adequately with their illness. Scales that were used in this study are among others: (1) a two-dimensional scale measuring the cancer patients needs for information, (2) a fear scale for cancer patients, (3) a loss of control scale for cancer patients, (4) a checklist measuring cancer patients' complaints, (5) a family support scale, (6) the Spielberger State Trait anxiety scale, (7) a self-esteem scale and (8) the Zung depression scale. The results show that whether or not patients actually make contact with other patients seems to be determined to an important extent by their feelings of uncertainty and anxiety. Apart from these factors, intrapersonal characteristics play an important role. In regard to patients' information-seeking behaviour, our study shows that this seems designed to alleviate feelings of anxiety and fear experienced by most of these patients.

The purpose of this article is to introduce some research which we have been doing on the situation, problems and coping processes of cancer patients. This research is part of a larger programme of psychosociological studies with cancer patients. Topics covered in

41

our research are: treatment related studies, information about cancer, and aspects of after-care.

From the list of references one can get an impression of our work.[1-12]

TREATMENT RELATED STUDIES

In relation to the side-effects of intrusive therapies, together with colleagues at other universities, we have developed a questionnaire to measure patients' physical and psychological complaints, the extent to which they can perform daily activities without help from others and further questions about their general well-being and use of medicines. This questionnaire, which can be regarded as a rough indicator of quality of life in cancer patients, has been used in several studies. In another study the psychosocial effects of two types of surgery for breast cancer (i.e. radical versus conservative treatment) have been compared. A more specific treatment study has been undertaken on certain antecedents of the adoption of the Moerman Diet, which is an alternative treatment and of particular public interest in The Netherlands. One of these antecedents was doctor–patient communication, a topic which also formed part of a more extensive study of the role of the family doctor at various stages of the patients' disease.

CANCER INFORMATION

This includes work on the patients' own needs for information after diagnosis, and we shall return to this later; and the evaluation both of the effects of public education about cancer and, more specifically, of an information brochure for breast cancer patients.

ASPECTS OF AFTER-CARE

For example, the social support derived from fellow sufferers, family, and medical specialists; and the activities and effects of self-help groups made up of ex-patients.

PROBLEMS

Our aim now is to focus on a particular project where we examined some of the problems which patients experience after they have had cancer diagnosed, their coping processes, and especially the help and support they receive from fellow sufferers. These problems include uncertainty, fear (and other negative feelings), loss of control, and threat to self-esteem. We assume that patients will want to see a reduction in these feelings of uncertainty and fear, will prefer to have control over this new situation and will want to maintain earlier levels of self-esteem. Our research looks at the way in which patients try to bring about these effects and, in particular, how they may use contact with fellow sufferers as a means of coping.

The two most important questions for research are: (1) what are the predisposing factors affecting the need for contact with fellow suffers, and how do patients go about making contact with them? and (2) is contact with fellow sufferers effective for cancer patients, in the sense that it leads to the reduction or solution of their problems?

The study which we carried out to try to answer these questions took a primarily sociopsychological approach as its point of departure, but before we expand on that, it may give a sharper flavour of our research if we describe the measuring instruments which we developed and a few of the results which they enabled us to obtain.

SAMPLE

We carried out interviews with two types of cancer patients in The Netherlands, for whom nationally organized after-care by fellow sufferers was available. Twenty-two medical specialists working in fifteen different medical centres across The Netherlands asked every patient with Hodgkin's disease and every breast cancer patient with whom they had contact at these centres, to co-operate in this investigation by being interviewed. Finally, 216 patients with Hodgkin's disease (or non-Hodgkin's lymphoma) and 282 breast cancer patients who had a mastectomy, were interviewed. Also, 122 ex-patients, who were working as volunteers in the after-care programme, were interviewed.

FIGURE 1. RESEARCH DESIGN

Groups		
Patients with Hodgkin's Disease (N = 216)	contact *with* fellow-suffer(s) *without* contact with fellow- sufferer(s)	109 107
Breast Cancer Patients who have had a mastectomy (N = 282)	contact *with* fellow-sufferer(s) *without* contact with fellow- sufferer(s)	109 126
Volunteers	ex-patients/volunteers with *Hodgkin's disease* ex-patients/volunteers with *breast cancer*	17 105

These interviews were conducted in the patients' homes during February and March 1982. One and a half years later the patients were interviewed again. The interviews were undertaken by 40 female interviewers with prior interviewing experience, who were specially trained in interviewing cancer patients. Each interview lasted approximately two hours and most of the questions were structured. Following the interview the patient completed the questionnaire at leisure.

MEASURING INSTRUMENTS

In Table 1 an overview of scales constructed in order to measure the problems experienced by cancer patients, is presented.

Most of these scales have a high reliability-coefficient. *Uncertainty* we take as experiencing a lack of information on areas which are important for the patient. So uncertainty implies a need for information. Uncertainty can be a very important form of stress for cancer patients. The patient has many questions about the disease and treatment, about self and feelings, and about interpersonal relations. Uncertainty can be measured by two subscales: one scale measures uncertainty about the prospects of the illness and treatment, the other measures uncertainty about the possibilities of obtaining help and getting solutions to problems related to illness and treatment.

TABLE 1. OVERVIEW OF CONSTRUCTED SCALES TO MEASURE PROBLEMS OF
CANCER PATIENTS

	Number of items	Cronbach's alpha	
		first measurement ($N = 498$)	second measurement ($N = 369$)
Uncertainty			
about the prospects of the illness and treatment	9	.93	.93
about possibilities of help and about getting solutions to problems related to the illness and treatment	8	.87	.88
Negative feelings			
Fear for the illness, the treatment and its consequences	11	.87	.88
Psychological complaints	8	.91	.90
Physical complaints	7	.82	.76
State anxiety (based on Spielberger)	18	.95	.94
Loneliness	5	.69	.66
Feelings of depression	10	.83	.83
Sleep disturbances	3	.71	.73
Loss of control	8	.77	.80
Self-esteem	4	.63	.69

The most commonly mentioned *negative feelings* in the literature are fear, anxiety and feelings of depression. We also used a measurement of loneliness and sleep disturbance and a list of physical and psychological complaints which we take to be an expression of the patient's emotional situation. *Loss of control* is defined as being unable to handle, manage or influence events. It can be a consequence of different events. For example, admission to hospital implies a submission to others' roles. The disease makes planning for the future difficult.

Physical aspects can also lead to an experienced loss of control, for example, in social contacts. The *threat to self-esteem* is considered an important stress reaction in cancer patients. Self-esteem can be related to one's feelings about one's own body; one's performance at work, in hobbies, domestic activities and to the quality of interpersonal relations. Cancer patients can easily suffer in all these respects. The different methods by which people may reduce these four, and other sources of stress, we term *"coping strategies"*. People can deal with a stressful situation better if they have more methods by which to manage it.

Two coping strategies in which we are particularly interested are information seeking and seeking the comfort and support of others. *Information* can reduce uncertainty, and may be sought from expert, professional sources, or failing those, through more informal channels, such as from fellow sufferers. Information sometimes will increase the feeling of having some control because patients may realize that they can do something about the situation. The *search for support and comfort* may also be directed at others who are in a similar situation to oneself. It can also be found through a partner, a good friend or nurse. The most important contribution is understanding and a feel for the situation. Support and comfort can reduce negative feelings, strengthen the feelings of control and increase self-esteem. With respect to this last coping strategy it is important to assess whether it is possible for the patient to seek support and comfort from his own family. That is why we developed a scale to measure the openness in the family to discussing the illness. The reliability of this scale is high: the Cronbach's alpha in the first measurement in .81, in the second .86.

RESULTS

The results indicate (Table 2) that both Hodgkin's and breast cancer patients felt most uncertain about the origin of their disease; and both groups also felt particularly uncertain about possible consequences of the disease, the results of treatment, and the purpose of treatment. With regard to some aspects of this type of uncertainty it is difficult to give the patient precise information (e.g. about the origin of the disease). On the other hand, there are questions which can be answered relatively easily, e.g. about side-effects, and the goal of the treatment, events surrounding the treatment and survival rates of the disease. By paying attention to these kinds of questions from patients, probably much uncertainty can be reduced. As can be noticed from Table 2, Hodgkin's patients expressed more uncertainty than the breast cancer patients sampled.

TABLE 2. UNCERTAINTY—SCALE 1: ABOUT THE PROSPECTS OF THE ILLNESS AND TREATMENT

Need (rather much or very much) information about:	Hodgkin (N = 216)	Breast cancer (N = 282)
1. The cause of their illness	77%	51%
2. Results of the treatment	56%	41%
3. Possible side-effects of the treatment	58%	38%
4. Possible results of their illness	58%	35%
5. The development of their illness	55%	36%
6. The goal/purpose of the treatment	51%	40%
7. Course of things around treatment	47%	33%
8. The survival-rates of the illness	46%	26%
9. Their present situation	39%	24%

In Table 3 we can also see that many patients are uncertain about the possibilities of help and about what they themselves can do to prevent and solve practical and psychological problems. About half of the Hodgkin's patients and one-third of the breast cancer patients need rather much or very much information about how they themselves can contribute to their health, e.g. by following a diet or doing exercises. It is noteworthy that so many patients need good educational materials and literature. Further, it can be noticed from

TABLE 3. UNCERTAINTY—SCALE 2: ABOUT THE POSSIBILITIES OF HELP AND ABOUT GETTING SOLUTIONS TO PROBLEMS RELATED TO THE ILLNESS AND TREATMENT

Need (rather much or very much) information about:	Hodgkin (N = 216)	Breast cancer (N = 282)
1. How to become or stay healthy (e.g. exercise, diet)	48%	34%
2. How to get good booklets or literature	44%	34%
3. Possibilities of getting first-aid if problems or questions about the illness	39%	27%
4. What they are allowed to do in their situation (e.g. work, hobby, eating and drinking)	33%	26%
5. How to talk with physician	29%	22%
6. How to talk about the illness with the people who are very close	29%	19%
7. Prosthesis (e.g. breast prosthesis, wigs)	12%	28%
8. How to find your way in the hospital	20%	18%

Table 3 that 28% of the patients with breast cancer need information about a prosthesis. We also interviewed ex-patients who worked as volunteers in giving after-care. According to these volunteers 82% of the patients need more information about a prosthesis.

Among negative feelings, fear that the disease would recur was prominent. There was also marked apprehension about undergoing new treatment, about being unable to do things any longer, becoming dependent, and of a complete decline. Hodgkin's patients also experienced a relatively strong apprehension of the side-effects of medicines. Tiredness was the most common physical or psychological complaint; followed by muscle-pains, worrying, nervousness, touchiness and feeling tense.

A majority of patients, particularly those with Hodgkin's disease, reported that they no longer felt "quite themselves", which is perhaps an indication of loss of control. More than two patients in five said that since or because of their disease they were no longer able to do what they used to do in their spare time or at work. More things worried them, and they had less grip on their emotions.

The threat to self-esteem was more a problem for breast cancer than for Hodgkin's patients. They felt themselves less physically attractive and as a result of the disease and its treatment they had less sexual contact with their partner. (In parentheses, we should complement this picture of patients' problems by reporting that in the interviews which we carried out, a majority also reported positive effects of cancer, in that they enjoyed life more than before.)

As far as the patients' coping strategies were concerned, many of them relied on talking themselves into better spirits when things were bad psychologically. Other reactions which occurred were: getting the whole business into perspective, actively looking for ways of improving the situation, shutting oneself off from problems, attending to other things, trying as quickly as possible to forget, and going to talk to one's partner. Only a few said that they went to talk to fellow sufferers in such circumstances. In fact their most important source of support was their partner, though very important support was also obtained from friends, relations, brothers and sisters. In hospital the patients obtained rather less support from the nursing staff, but an important measure of support from their specialist. Outside the hospital only one in three considered their family doctor an important supportive figure. Finally, about one in four revealed that they had obtained important support from one or more fellow sufferers.

By "contact with fellow sufferers" we understand a form of personal contact which people have with one or more patients or ex-patients with the same illness, through correspondence, or face-to-face, or telephone conversations about problems and experiences. Just over one-half of our sample had at some at some time made contact with fellow sufferers.

A wide range of factors was associated with the need for contact with fellow sufferers. What was particularly clear was a relation between that need and uncertainty and directing one's attention to obtaining more information. In Hodgkin's patients this consisted, in particular, of uncertainty about the prospects of the disease and treatment (connected perhaps with the "mysterious" character of the disease); and in breast cancer patients of uncertainty about the possibilities of help and relief, for example, information about where to get good educational materials and information.

The factors associated with *actually* making contact with fellow sufferers are above all concerned with other coping strategies. For example, the breast cancer patients who made contact were people who are inclined to seek information and support from others and are not inclined to "give up" in stressful situations. The corresponding Hodgkin's patients were people who above all perceived themselves as having control over what happens to them. In this case they see themselves as having the ability to influence the course of their disease, and this perception is strongly connected to the search for fellow sufferers. Of course we realize the importance of describing the eventual *effects* of contact with fellow sufferers, on the problems experienced by cancer patients. At this moment, however, we are in the analysis phase of this study.

DISCUSSION

How do we make sense of our research and the findings at a theoretical level? We have deliberately left this until now in order to underline its interpretative significance.

We have been looking at the problems and possible solutions which people face when, at a particular moment in their life, they are suddenly confronted with the fact that they have cancer. We can conceptualize the process in terms of two sociopsychological theories—social comparison theory and attribution theory.

It is a fundamental proposition of social comparison theory that in cases of uncertainty, which we have seen to be an essential feature of the patients' experience, people will first try to reduce their uncertainty by means of as much objective information as possible—"hard facts"—from the professionals, for example, who are treating them. If objective information cannot be obtained in this way—and we have seen that this is the experience of many patients—they will seek it from others and preferably from people like themselves. Thus the theory would predict that the uncertain cancer patient will eventually seek out fellow sufferers so that he or she can clarify ideas about the disease and its treatment and about possible solutions to the problems.

Social comparison theory also proposes that people will seek the company of comparable others if they are afraid. Such contact will reduce fear, through mutual support, trust, confirmation and encouraging one another. It can also enable people to evaluate their feelings of fear; that is, by comparing themselves with people in the same situation, they can find out whether or not their feelings are "normal". You can say that somebody who is uncertain wants to be able to predict his situation; but he will also want to influence his situation as much as possible. In other words he wants control. Attribution theory assumes that people attach causes and intentions to events in order to get control; they are continually engaged in looking for links between causes and effects so that they can, among other things, get an idea of how their behaviour can influence their situation. For example: "If I stick to my special diet, then I still have a good chance."

With regard to various aspects of the disease, people can make very different attributions. For example, we found that two-thirds of all the patients we interviewed reported that they thought they could influence the course of the disease (they make an internal attribution). We also found that only one out of eight patients thinks that the illness is caused by himself or his life-style: so, with respect to this, more external attributions are made. We have an indication that the way people make certain attributions influences the coping strategies they choose, as well as their health behaviour. For example, we found that Hodgkin's patients who attribute the cause of their illness to themselves or their life-style are less inclined to forget their problems, are less inclined to direct their attention towards other things if confronted with problems but are more inclined to talk to others about their problems (for instance with relatives and friends).

With respect to health behaviour, we found that patients who attribute the cause of their illness to themselves or their life-style and at the same time feel that they may influence the course of their illness, pay more attention to their food and diet. On the contrary, patients who also attribute the cause of their illness to themselves but *do not* feel that they may influence the future development of their illness, do not bother about their food or diet. With regard to contact with fellow sufferers, we found especially that those Hodgkin's patients who do make contact, make internal attributions with respect to the cause and course of their disease.

We hypothesize that the strategy of seeking contact with a fellow sufferer can lead to a reduction of uncertainty and negative feelings, such as fear, but can also lead to reduction of feelings of loss of control. Social comparison with somebody who is a living example of how to get back to normal life again could give the patient the feeling that he or she can influence the situation and have control.

Finally, to round off the story, we would like to make two concluding remarks.

First, we can conclude that help, given by a volunteer or ex-patient, is not a panacea for all patients. About half of the Hodgkin's patients and one-third of the breast cancer patients need "rather much" or "very much" information about how others, who are in the same circumstances, react to their illness and treatment.

Second, we found that there is still a relatively large group of patients who have difficulty in getting into contact with a fellow sufferer. For this purpose we decided to produce a book in which information is provided about the possible problems and coping strategies of cancer patients.

This is written for patients and their relatives and is especially based on the diaries of cancer patients. We believe that such a book can help patients to make social comparisons.

REFERENCES

1. Pruyn, J. F. A., Maguire, P. and Haes, de J. C. J. M. (1981) Two methods of measuring some aspects of quality of life. *Proceedings of the Second EORTC Quality of Life Workshop*, Copenhagen, November 1981 (internal report), pp. 52–55.
2. Pruyn, J. F. A. and Haes, de J. C. J. M. (1981) Comparison of two instruments for measuring the quality of life in cancer patients. *Proceedings of the Second EORTC Quality of Life Workshop*, Copenhagen, November 1981 (internal report), pp. 69–91.

3. Pruyn, J. F. A. (1983) Coping with stress in cancer patients. *Patient Education and Counseling,* **5** (2), 57–62.
4. Siero, S., Kok, G. J. and Pruyn, J. F. A. (1984) Effects of public education about breast cancer and breast self-examination. *Social Science and Medicine,* **18** (10), 881–888.
5. Pruyn, J. F. A. and Jonkers, R. (1984) Reach to recovery: evaluation of an educational brochure for women with mastectomy. *Journal of the Institute of Health Education,* **22** (3), 92–99.
6. Pruyn, J. F. A., Rijckman, R. M., Brunschot, van C. J. M. and Borne, van den H. W. (1985) Cancer patients' personality characteristics, physician-patient communication, and the adoption of the Moerman diet. *Social Science and Medicine,* **20,** 841–847.
7. Pruyn, J. F. A. and Heuvel, van den W. J. A. (in press) Anxiety and social comparison in cancer patients. In: *Stress and Anxiety,* vol. 11. Spielberger, C. D., Sarason, I. G. and Defares, P. B. (eds), Hemisphere: New York.
8. Pruyn, J. F. A. and Borne, van den H. W. (1985) Self-care in cancer patients, *Quality of Life in Cancer,* Beckmann, J. (ed), Raven Press (in the EORTC Monograph series).
9. Vink, A., Pruyn, J. F. A. and Borne, van den H. W. (in press) A study on self-help groups. *Proceedings of the Third World Congress of "Reach to Recovery".* Israël Cancer Association.
10. Molleman, E., Pruyn, J. F. A. and Knippenberg, van A. F. M. (in press) Social comparison processes among cancer patients. *British Journal of Social Psychology.*
11. Jonkers, R., Pruyn, J. F. A. and The, S. K. Mastectomy versus breast saving therapy: some psychosocial considerations. Submitted for publication.
12. Borne, van den H. W., Pruyn, J. F. A. and Mey, de K. (in press) Help by fellow patients. In: *Coping with cancer stress,* Stoll, B. A. (ed), Martinus Nijhoff, Dordrecht (The Netherlands).

SECTION THREE

Psychological Responses To Diagnosis and Treatment

Mastectomy versus Breast Conservation: Psychological Effects of Patient Choice of Treatment

J. J. ASHCROFT,* S. J. LEINSTER** and P. D. SLADE[1]

ABSTRACT

Women with early breast cancer were treated with either mastectomy (plus reconstruction for some patients) or lumpectomy and radiotherapy. Where possible a choice of treatments was offered. Psychological effects were investigated using tests of anxiety, depression, body satisfaction, self-esteem, sociability, and life change. Patients were also interviewed to assess degree of concern about the disease, their appearance, and the treatment. The major difference between groups was in the degree of concern about appearance. Those women who expressed a high degree of concern about maintaining a complete body image opted for either lumpectomy, or, if a mastectomy was necessary, for a breast reconstruction. It is suggested that women in this study did not suffer from many of the symptoms reported for breast cancer patients (depression, lessened self-esteem, body dissatisfaction, and social withdrawal) because in nearly all cases the gross physical change usually associated with early breast cancer treatment could be avoided.

* Sub-department of Clinical Psychology, New Medical School, Ashton Street, P.O. Box 147, Liverpool L69 3BX, UK

** Department of Surgery, Royal Liverpool Hospital, Prescot Street, Liverpool L7 8XP, UK

All authors are members of the University of Liverpool, and their research is funded by the Cancer Research Campaign.

Address for reprints: Jennifer Ashcroft, Ph.D., Sub-department of Clinical Psychology, New Medical School, Ashton Street, P.O. Box 147, Liverpool L69 3BX.

The authors wish to thank the hospital staff who co-operated with this study, and those women who participated in the project.

The traditional treatment for breast cancer has been mastectomy. Yet the psychological effects of both having a serious illness and being the subject of a mutilating operation have been little investigated until the last fifteen years. Now it would appear that particular difficulties and patterns of emotional and social response are beginning to emerge. Depression is the most common effect of mastectomy,[1, 2] often accompanied by anxiety.[3, 4] These responses are persistent, and where long-term studies have been conducted, have been shown to persist well into the first and even the second year following the mastectomy.[5-7] There are, predictably, other psychological and social responses reported, such as anger,[8] difficulties in performing tasks around the home,[9] and in returning to work,[10] and problems with adapting to a different body image.[11] There is also reported concern about loss of femininity,[12] general marital and sexual problems,[13, 14] lowered self-esteem,[15] and an inability to function socially.[16]

In reviews of the literature on psychological effects of breast cancer,[17, 18] the studies cited are nearly always concerned with one mode of treatment, mastectomy. A control group may be absent, or more often consists of patients with benign breast lumps,[19] or patients with totally different diseases,[20] or people with no special pathology, population controls.[21] There exist, therefore, very few examples of research comparing psychological effects of mastectomy with other forms of treatment for breast cancer, particularly with operations which conserve the breast. There is growing concern about the need to remove the whole breast in order to treat the cancer. Trials have been conducted comparing the success (in terms of rate of local recurrence of the cancer and overall survival rate) of various forms of breast cancer treatment.[22, 23] Survival rates for conservative treatment, removal of malignant lump rather than the whole breast, appear in some reports to be comparable to mastectomy as a treatment.[24, 25] It would seem likely, therefore, that conservative surgery could increasingly become the treatment of choice. However, there are very few studies concerned with comparing psychological effects of these two treatments. Atkins *et al.*[26] found little difference between the two procedures, but this conclusion was based on very limited psychological testing. A more recent study by Sanger and Reznikoff[27] compared psychological effects of breast saving techniques with mastectomy. They found that the women who had conservative surgery showed greater intactness of their external body boundaries and less change in overall body satisfaction than women in the mastectomy group. There were no significant differences between the two groups on measures of body anxiety, general psychological adjustment or marital satisfaction. It was suggested that all the women were experiencing high concern about their bodies as a result of the disease, rather than because of the operation, and that this might account for similar body anxiety across the two groups. It was also suggested that the mastectomy group was representative of that population which adapts well to surgery; all agreed without question to the mastectomy suggested by the surgeon, and were sufficiently emotionally stable to agree to participate in the study, which entailed two hours of psychological testing. Finally, the authors concluded that surgical procedure had no differential effect on marital satisfaction.

The purpose of the present study was to further investigate the psychological impact of mastectomy and of more conservative surgery as treatments for breast cancer. As yet very little is known about the differential effects of these two procedures. Psychological tests used in previous studies have been narrow in range when compared to the more extensive testing used with the studies concerned primarily with mastectomy patients. Testing over time, with questionnaires given before and after surgery, and at long-term follow-up, has not been done. Finally, little account has been taken of the effect of patient choice of operation. Presumably if results so far indicate that both surgical procedures might be equally effective, it is possible that there might be scope for the patient having a deciding role in choice of operation, and this could well have an effect on psychological well-being. The present investigation was therefore designed to incorporate the above factors, a broad range of tests and interviews, repeated over many occasions, with patient choice of operation as a further factor to be investigated in elucidating psychological effects of mastectomy versus conservative surgery.

METHOD

The present study reports on 31 women who underwent some form of breast surgery. In accordance with the policy of our unit, women with proven breast cancer were treated by either mastectomy or lumpectomy with radiotherapy. Where mastectomy was considered essential, women were offered reconstruction of the breast where it was technically feasible.

Women with breast problems were routinely seen when they

presented at the clinic and were invited to participate in the present study. Subjects were from a wide range of social classes and covered a wide age range (21–70 years). Many of the patients did not have serious breast pathology and after examination (and mammography if appropriate) were discharged from further attendance at the unit. Younger women with clinical fibroadenomas underwent breast biopsy as day cases. The patients reported on in this study were those who were admitted to hospital for treatment.

This unit is participating in the CRC Breast Conservation Trial. Patients who fulfilled the entry criteria for the trial were offered entry into the trial or the alternative of choosing between lumpectomy and mastectomy outside the trial.

Several groups were therefore generated. Group 1 comprised those patients in whom, on surgical grounds, mastectomy was considered to be the only treatment option. To those offered a choice there were three options. Firstly, they could choose to enter the medical trial where the decision to either have a mastectomy (Group 2) or a lumpectomy (Group 3) was a matter of random allocation. The second option that could be chosen was mastectomy (Group 4) and the third option was lumpectomy (Group 5). With Group 6, it was considered inappropriate to offer mastectomy for a variety of reasons, and so lumpectomy was performed. The patients in Group 7 consisted of women for whom a mastectomy was decided without patient choice (as with Group 1) but who had opted for immediate breast reconstruction (the same day as the mastectomy). Group 8 consisted of women who had a mastectomy before the present study began and who were now being given a breast reconstruction. And finally, some subjects were undergoing investigative operations on breast lumps which proved to be benign, and these women constituted Group 9.

The largest group was Group 1 (n = 7). There were five patients in Group 5, four patients in each of Groups 4, 7 and 9, two patients in each of Groups 2, 3 and 6, and one patient in Group 8. There was no significant difference in social class or marital status between groups, but there was a significant difference in age ($p < 0.0097$). Where the breast lumps were benign (Group 9) or small enough to warrant lumpectomy with no choice of mastectomy (Group 6) or where reconstructions were chosen (Groups 7 and 8), patients tended to be younger (below 45 years of age). The other groups consisted of women older than this, with Groups 1 and 2 having the oldest patients (a mean age of 62 and 63 years respectively).

Psychological adjustment was gauged by a series of tests given to subjects on four possible occasions: (i) when the women first presented at clinic for medical assessment, (ii) the day before the operation, (iii) two days and then (iv) three months following surgery. Patients were also interviewed on the occasion of the second and third testing sessions (the day before and two days after their operation).

TESTS AND MEASURES

Subjects were given a battery of tests when first seen. This battery was designed to be completed by the patient herself in a time period of approximately 35 minutes.

Depression and Anxiety

Measures of depression and anxiety were obtained using the Leeds scales[28] which consist of self-rating scales based on the Wakefield SAD Inventory with added items. Using these scales it is possible to measure the severity of depressive illness and anxiety neurosis (with the Leeds Depression Specific scale and Leeds Anxiety Specific scale respectively). The Leeds Depression General scale and Anxiety General scale can be used to indicate whether a person is in a pure depressive or a pure anxiety state, or alternatively whether the patient exhibits both depressive and anxiety symptoms.

Additional measures of anxiety were taken with the Spielberger State-Trait Anxiety Inventory.[29] The State scale consists of 20 statements that ask people to describe how they feel at a particular moment in time, and the Trait scale also has 20 statements concerned with how people generally feel. The Trait scale may be used to assess anxiety proneness and the State scale may be used as an indicator of transitory anxiety.

Body Satisfaction

The General scale consists of 16 body parts which the patient is asked to rate on a measure of satisfaction between 1 (very satisfied) and 7 (very unsatisfied).

There are also similar measures of satisfaction relating

specifically to the breasts. The patient is asked to rate degree of satisfaction with the size, shape, general appearance, and comfort of the breast area. This scale was designed specifically for the present study.

Social Adaptability

Watson and Friend[30] have developed two scales to measure social-evaluative anxiety, the Fear of Negative Evaluation scale (FNE) and the Social Avoidance and Distress scale (SAD). They found that people who scored highly on the SAD scale tended to avoid social interactions, preferred to work alone, talked little and were generally worried and lacked confidence in social relationships. Those high in FNE became nervous in evaluative situations and worked hard to gain approval. Both scales were used in the present study to measure possible difference in these areas between groups.

Marital Satisfaction

The Locke and Wallace Marital-Adjustment Test[31] consists of a 15 item self-administered questionnaire designed to give a measure of marital harmony, and covers a wide range of subjects, pertaining, for example, to sexual relations; handling of family finances; hobbies; and ways of dealing with in-laws.

Self-esteem

A measure of self-esteem was obtained with the PERI[32] scales, eight questions which deal with, for example, the frequency with which a person feels self-confident, or feels useless; whether the person feels they have anything to be proud of; whether the person is satisfied with themselves, and so on.

Life Events

It has been suggested[33] that the occurrence of life events such as moving house, changing job, death of a close relative, may be related to the onset of disease and perhaps also to the ways in which the person adapts to the diseased state. The frequency and type of major life events was therefore monitored in the present study, using the Holmes and Rahe[34] Social Readjustment Rating scale. This requires the person to indicate which of a given list of life events has happened to them (in the present study, in the course of the year prior to the questionnaire being filled in). An additional category was added to the questionnaire where the patient could add any major life events which they had experienced but which were not on the list (for example, finding a breast lump).

The batch of questionnaires described above was given to each patient either when they first presented with a breast problem at clinic or, where they were not seen at clinic (or where they had not wished to do the questionnaires at clinic) they were given the day before the operation. Understandably perhaps, not all patients were willing to spend time answering a large number of questions the day before surgery. For those who refused to do the whole battery (just a few women) the Spielberger tests of anxiety and the Leeds scales (anxiety and depression) were given.

Two days after the operation the Spielberger State scale of anxiety and the Leeds scales were again given. Three months following surgery the full batch of questionnaires were sent to the patient to complete and return. A follow-up after one year is also planned, but, as yet, data are not available on this final testing period.

The Adjustment Questionnaire

In addition to the above battery of tests an additional questionnaire was sent, devised specifically for the present study, which asked direct questions about life following the operation. All patients except those with benign lumps (Group 9) were sent this. The questionnaire deals with three areas. The first part is concerned with activity level (for example, can the women do domestic tasks or indulge in leisure activities as she did before the operation?; has she resumed her job?; are these activities as easy to perform as before?). The second area is concerned with relationships with husband, family and friends. And the final part of the questionnaire is concerned with thoughts about health and general well-being (a retrospective view of treatment; present feelings; and hopes for the future).

Interviews

The day before surgery an extensive interview was given in addition to the standard tests described earlier. Each patient was invited to talk about her problems, including, where relevant, any difficulties about choosing between type of operation. In addition, for all groups except Group 9 (investigative surgery) the patient was asked to give a number (between 1 and 10) to indicate degree of concern about each of three problem areas. The first area was the disease itself, the fact that the patient had cancer; the second area was the patient's appearance, with any concern the woman might have about the way she would look after surgery and the importance of the look of her breasts; and the third area dealt with feelings about being in hospital and having to undergo medical treatment which included an operation.

Two days following surgery the patient was again seen, given the relevant questionnaires as described above, and was the subject of a largely unstructured interview designed to explore the patient's thoughts and experiences since the operation.

TESTING AND INTERVIEW PROCEDURE

Women were seen individually by the first author for tests and interviews. The first testing period, at the clinic, lasted only 30 to 40 minutes, the time taken to fill in the full batch of questionnaires.

The day before the operation the patient was asked if she wished to participate further in the study. If she agreed she was first interviewed usually for at least one hour. Following the interview the patient was left with the batch of questionnaires to fill in herself.

During the post-operative interview most women were, understandably, tired, and therefore this talk tended to be brief, no more than 30 minutes. Just a few questionnaires were then given to the patient to complete.

Tests were sent by post to the patient after three months, although she was also invited to contact the first author if she felt the need for extra help, or if she simply wanted to talk about her experiences.

RESULTS

Analysis of variance was used to compare scores between each of the nine groups, for each test given, on each occasion the test was given (Analysis 1).

Further analyses were conducted by joining some of the original nine groups to form new categories. So, instead of having nine separate groups, in Analysis 2, Groups 1, 2 and 4 were combined to form a single group of women who had mastectomies (Group M); Groups 3, 5 and 6 became a single lumpectomy group (Group L); and Groups 7 and 8 constituted the mastectomy and reconstruction group (Group MR). Therefore the three new groups M, L and MR, represented the three different types of operation performed. An analysis of variance was again used to compare scores between these three groups for each test given, on each occasion it was given.

In Analysis 3 the original nine groups were divided in yet a different way, in terms of choice of operation. Those patients who were given a choice of treatment (Groups 2, 3, 4 and 5) were considered as a single group (Group C), and those who had no choice (Groups 1, 6, 7 and 8) became Group NC. An analysis of variance was then used to compare scores between these two groups for each test given, on each occasion it was given.

Depression and Anxiety

With the Spielberger tests of anxiety, there was no significant difference between groups on any occasion the test was given. This was true for all of the three major analyses described above. All groups showed some degree of anxiety pre-operatively, but scores approximated the norms for general surgical patients; very high anxiety scores did not occur at any time of testing.

With the Leeds Scales there was no significant difference between the groups in Analysis 1 and 2. The degree of anxiety and depression was within the range for normals (scoring between 0 and 7 on the 0–18 scale) rather than psychiatrically sick patients (a score high on the 0–18 scale).

There was a significant difference ($p < 0.05$) between Group C and NC (Analysis 3) with the Leeds Scale of general anxiety, when this test was given the day before operation. Group C ($N = 13$) had a mean score of 7.2 (s.d. $= 3.5$) and Group NC ($N = 13$) had a mean score of 4.1 (s.d. $= 3.5$). With this scale, the higher the score the greater the anxiety. It would seem, therefore, that those patients who could choose between operations showed greater anxiety than those who could not. This difference did not occur at any other time pre- or post-operatively and therefore could possibly reflect problems in trying to choose between operations. This does not mean, however, that giving such a choice is necessarily detrimental to the patient; the degree of anxiety for both groups was still relatively small (the "cut-off" around a score of 6 to 7 provides the best indicator between health and sickness on this scale, which ranges from 0 to 18).

With Analysis 3 there was also a significant difference ($p < 0.05$) with the Leeds Scale score which differentiates between depressive and anxiety states, when this test was given three months postoperatively. The mean score for Group C was −2.1 (s.d.=1.7) and the mean score for Group NC was 0.2 (s.d.=1.7). With the scale, a score below −4 indicates a "pure anxiety" state. So although there was a difference between groups on this measure, both show some symptoms of anxiety and depression. However, the other scores on the Leeds Scale show the degree of anxiety and depression to be very small, within the range for normals.

Body Satisfaction

With the General Scale there was no significant difference between groups (with all three analyses) on any occasion the test was given. Scores approximated those of a normal population.

With the body satisfaction measures relating specifically to the breasts, again there was no significant difference between the groups in any of the analyses, when this test was given the day before surgery or at any time after surgery. The women were generally satisfied with the breast region. However, when this test was given at clinic (at the first possible testing session) there was a significant difference between groups on all three analyses. With Analysis 1 the significant difference in scores was $p < 0.05$; with Analysis 2, $p < 0.05$; with Analysis 3, $p < 0.01$. However, it is notable that far fewer women wished to participate in the study at this early stage when they first presented at clinic; and only seven subjects were willing to fill in the questionnaires then. Of these seven, two of the women had very low body satisfaction (one had a compulsory mastectomy, the other had a compulsory mastectomy and reconstruction). Thus the significant difference between groups might perhaps be considered something of an artifact here, caused by two extreme scores for two women, when the total number of subjects was low.

Social Adaptability, Marital Satisfaction and Self-esteem

There were no significant differences between groups with any of the analyses. Generally, scores approximated those for a normal population.

Life Events

There was no significant difference between groups in Analysis 2 and 3. However, in Analysis 1, where patients were seen the day before operation, there was a significant difference ($p < 0.05$) between the nine groups for number of life events reported. The lowest number of reported events occurred in the trial mastectomy group (mean= 2 s.d.=0) and trial lumpectomy group (mean=2 s.d.=0). The mean for the compulsory mastectomy group was 2.7 events (s.d.=1.2). Those who chose lumpectomy reported a mean number of 3 events (s.d.=1.41). Patients who had compulsory lumpectomy, compulsory mastectomy plus reconstruction, and reconstruction only, each reported a mean of 4 life events (s.d.=0, 2, 0 respectively). Those who had investigative surgery (for benign lumps) reported a mean of 4.25 events (s.d.=0.95), and those who chose a mastectomy reported a mean of 5.5 life events (s.d.=0.58). These figures are reported to make it clear that there is no trend for type of operation, or choice of operation, or severity of disease, to be differentially associated with reported number of life events experienced in the previous year. Although there are significant differences between groups the figures show that the mean number of life events only varied between 2 and 5.5. These are still relatively small numbers when it is considered that it is possible with this questionnaire to pick dozens of wide ranging life events (for example, taking a vacation; change in number of family get-togethers; marriage). It is worth noting that it is possible with this questionnaire to weight the severity of life events, and when this was done there were no significant differences between groups.

The Adjustment Questionnaire

This questionnaire was given three months after surgery. There were no significant differences between groups on the sections concerned with activity level or relationships. With the section on health and general well-being, there was no significant difference between groups for Analysis 2 and 3; however, there was a significant difference ($p<0.05$) for Analysis 1. As with the body satisfaction (breast area) discussed earlier, this result was largely an artifact caused by a low number of subjects in some groups, who had extreme scores. Generally, post-operative adjustment was good for all patients in all groups.

Concern about Appearance, Disease and the Operation

The results for concern (on a scale from 1 to 10) for each of these three topics discussed in interview are given in Table 1.

There was a significant difference ($p<0.001$) between the nine groups in Analysis 1, in concern about appearance. There was also a

TABLE 1. ANALYSES 1, 2 AND 3 FOR THE THREE MAJOR AREAS OF CONCERN

		Appearance	Disease	Operation
For Total	Mean	4.93	6.56	4.11
Population	S.D.	3.16	2.76	2.89
	(N)	27	27	27
Analysis 1				
	F Value	5.94	1.64	1.20
	Sig.	0.0009	0.19	0.35
Analysis 2				
Type	F Value	13.24	0.95	0.63
Op.	Sig.	0.0001	0.40	0.54
Analysis 3				
Choice	F Value	0.06	0.89	1.28
Op.	Sig.	0.81	0.36	0.27

significant difference ($p<0.001$) in concern over appearance between the three groups in Analysis 2. Table 2 shows the mean and standard deviation scores for the groups in Analysis 1, and Table 3 gives these scores for Analysis 2. It is clear from these figures that the women who had a mastectomy with reconstruction were less concerned about their appearance than those who either had a lumpectomy, or those who decided to have a reconstruction following a mastectomy.

TABLE 2. MEAN SCORES AND STANDARD DEVIATIONS FOR GROUPS IN ANALYSIS 1 FOR RATING ON CONCERN ABOUT APPEARANCE (ON A SCALE FROM 1 TO 10)

Group	Mean	S.D.	N
1	2.4	1.5	7
2	3.5	3.5	2
3	2.5	2.1	2
4	2.7	2.2	4
5	7.8	1.3	5
6	6.5	4.9	2
7	8.3	1.3	4
8	8.0	0	1

$F = 5.938$ Sig. $= 0.0009$

TABLE 3. MEAN SCORES AND STANDARD DEVIATIONS FOR GROUPS IN ANALYSIS 2 FOR RATING ON CONCERN ABOUT APPEARANCE (ON A SCALE FROM 1 TO 10)

Groups	Mean	S.D.	N
Mastectomy	2.7	1.9	13
Lumpectomy	6.3	3.1	9
Mastectomy and reconstruction	8.2	1.1	5

$F = 13.235$ Sig. $= 0.0001$

Given the highly significant differences between groups in Analysis 1 and 2, it may at first seem peculiar that there was no significant difference between the "Choice" and "No choice" groups in Analysis 3, with concern about appearance. This is largely because Group 7 (compulsory mastectomy plus immediate reconstruction) and Group 8 (reconstruction) were both included in the "No choice" category on the grounds that removal of the whole breast was considered necessary and lumpectomy was never deemed a viable alternative. However, a reconstruction was offered, and the patient could *choose* to accept this option, and it might therefore be considered appropriate to include these women in the "Choice" group; if appearance was important to them they could choose to remain as physically intact as possible. It is clear from the scores given in Table 2 that the inclusion of groups 7 and 8 in Group NC in Analysis 3 led to the insignificant differences between Groups C and NC.

DISCUSSION

There are two major findings from this study. Firstly, patients in all groups showed good psychosocial adaptation to the disease and to treatment. Many studies in the literature report high levels of anxiety, and prolonged anxiety and depression which may continue for many months or even years after surgery. At this stage in the analysis it is possible to conclude that there is no severe depression and anxiety up to three months after surgery. Testing at later periods has started to be conducted and, so far, results show psychological adaptation to treatment continues up to at least one year after surgery.

Secondly, there was a major difference between groups in degree of concern about appearance, that is, the importance of maintaining an intact body image. It was apparent from interview, that for some women, being able to remain as whole as possible (by choosing conservative surgery or a reconstruction after a medically necessary mastectomy) was of paramount importance to psychological well-being. All women who chose a lumpectomy or a reconstruction reported that they would have experienced considerable distress if they had lost a breast or if their physical appearance had altered greatly. Without exception they reported that they thought they could cope with the cancer knowing that physical disfigurement would be minimal. The results therefore indicate that, given alternative treatments for breast cancer, the best predictor of a positive psychological outcome is via a pre-operative interview in which the patient is given information about possible treatments and outcome and where the woman is offered help in aiding her own choice of treatment. It would seem that where concern about appearance is high she is likely to choose a more conservative operation or, given a mastectomy, a reconstruction. This is likely to be the case even though these women express concern about the disease itself which is as great as the concern expressed by those women who opt for a mastectomy, who forgo the opportunity to have the less mutilating operation.

From verbal reports during the interview prior to surgery, it would seem that, in terms of psychological well-being, there is no single treatment which is clearly "best". Although being able to choose lumpectomy was crucially important for some women, those who chose mastectomy often reported that they would have been distressed by receiving the alternative treatment. This was for a variety of reasons, for example, wanting to avoid radiotherapy, or the prolonged contact with hospital that attending for radiotherapy necessarily involves. Being able to choose their own treatment was therefore important for the women in this study. If they had been randomly allocated to the two major treatments, it seems probable that psychological adaptation would have been less good.

CONCLUSIONS

It is notable that the women in this study did not suffer from abnormally high levels of depression and anxiety; levels were those that might be expected for a normal person undergoing a stressful event, as discussed earlier in the context of results with the Leeds Scales. With the Spielberger tests of anxiety, results were in accord with this, as scores approximated the norm for general surgical patients. The various treatments did not result in any differences between groups for most of the variables studied. Generally patients' scores were not distinguishable from those of a normal population. So, for example, marital satisfaction, self-esteem, sociability, were typical of that of the "average" woman. It is suggested that the women in this study did not suffer from many of the symptoms reported for breast cancer patients (e.g. marked depression, loss of self-esteem, social withdrawal) because whenever possible a choice of operation was offered and the psychological distress involved in the gross physical change usually involved with a mastectomy was avoided. The results are generally in accord with those reported by Sanger and Reznikoff[27] for mastectomy and breast conservation procedures, but go further in suggesting that patient choice of operation is of importance. The best predictor of good psychological adjustment following breast cancer treatment is to establish, before operation, the patient's need to maintain a complete body image and, whenever possible, to adjust treatment accordingly.

REFERENCES

1. Anstice, E. (1970) The emotional operation 1. *Nursing Times*, **66**, 837–838.
2. Goldsmith, H. S. and Alday, E. S. (1971) Role of surgeon in the rehabilitation of the breast cancer patient. *Cancer*, **28**, 1672–1675.
3. Roberts, M. M., Furnival, I. G. and Forrest, A. P. M. (1972) The morbidity of mastectomy. *British Journal of Surgery*, **59**, 301–302.

4. Schoenberg, B. and Carr, A. C. (1970) Loss of external organs : Limb amputation, mastectomy and disfiguration. In: Schoenberg, B., Carr, A. C., Peretz, D. and Kutsher, A. H. (Eds.), *Loss and Grief: Psychological Management in Medical Practice*, New York: Columbia University Press.

5. Lee, E. C. G. and Maguire, G. P. (1975) Emotional distress in patients attending a breast clinic. *British Journal of Surgery*, **62**, 162.

6. Maguire, P. (1978) Psychiatric problems after mastectomy. In: Brand, P. C. and Van Keep, P. A. (Eds.) *Breast Cancer: Psycho-social Aspects of Early Detection and Treatment*. MTP Press, Lancaster.

7. Morris, T. (1979) Psychological adjustment to mastectomy. *Cancer Treatment Reviews*, **6**, 41.

8. Robbins, G. F. (1973) Nursing management of patients with breast tumours. In: Behnke, H. D. (Ed.) *Guidelines for Comprehensive Nursing Care in Cancer*, Springer, New York.

9. Bard, M. and Dyk, R. B. (1956) The psychodynamic significance of beliefs regarding the cause of serious illness. *The Psychoanalytic Review*, **43**, 146.

10. Morris, T., Greer, H. S. and White, P. (1977) Psychological and social adjustment to mastectomy. *Cancer*, **40**, 2381.

11. Buls, J. G., Jones, I. H., Bennett, R. C. and Chan, D. P. S. (1976) Women's attitudes to mastectomy for breast cancer. *The Medical Journal of Australia*, **2**, 336.

12. Ray, C. (1977) Psychological implications of mastectomy. *British Journal of Social and Clinical Psychology*, **16**, 373.

13. Jamison, K. R., Wellisch, D. K. and Pasnau, R. O. (1978) Psychosocial aspects of mastectomy: 1. The woman's perspective. *American Journal of Psychiatry*, **135**, 432.

14. Anstice, E. (1970) Coping after a mastectomy. *Nursing Times*, **66**, 882–883.

15. Polivy, J. (1977) Psychological effects of mastectomy on a woman's feminine self-concept. *Journal of Nervous and Mental Disease*, **164**, 77.

16. Burdick, D. (1975) Rehabilitation of the breast cancer patient. *Cancer*, **36**, 645.

17. Meyerowitz, B. E. (1980) Psychosocial correlates of breast cancer and its treatment. *Psychological Bulletin*, **87**, 108.

18. Ray, C. (1980) Psychological aspects of early breast cancer and its treatment. In: Rachman, S. (Ed.), *Contributions to Medical Psychology*, vol. 2. Pergamon Press.

19. Maguire, G. P., Lee, E. G., Bevington, D. J., Kuchemann, C., Crabtree, R. J. and Cornell, C. E. (1978) Psychiatric problems in the first year after mastectomy. *British Medical Journal*, **i**, 963.

20. Weisman, A. D. and Worden, J. W. (1976) The existential plight in cancer: significance of the first 100 days. *International Journal of Psychiatric Medicine*, **7**, 1.

21. Craig, T. J. Comstock, G. W. and Geiser, P. B. (1974) The quality of survival in breast cancer: a case control comparison. *Cancer*, **33**, 1451.

22. Halnan, K. E. (1979) Place and role of radiotherapy after surgery for breast cancer. In: Bonadonna, G., Mathe, G. and Solomon, S. E. (Eds.), *Adjuvant Therapies and Markers of Post-surgical Minimal Residual Disease*. Springer, New York.

ery.

23. Hayward, J. L. (1977) The Guy's trial of treatments of early breast cancer. *World Journal of Surgery*, **1**, 314.
24. Mustakallio, S. (1972) Conservative treatment of breast carcinoma—review of 25 years follow-up. *Clinical Radiology*, **23**, 110.
25. Rissanen, P. (1969) A comparison of conservative and radical surgery combined with radiotherapy in the treatment of stage 1 carcinoma of the breast. *British Journal of Radiology*, **42**, 423.
26. Atkins, H., Hayward, J., Klugman, D. and Wayte, A. (1972) Treatment of breast cancer: a report after ten years of a clinical trial. *British Medical Journal*, **20**, 423.
27. Sanger, C. K. and Reznikoff, M. (1981) A comparison of the psychological effects of breast saving procedures with the modified radical mastectomy. *Cancer*, **48**, 2341.
28. Snaith, R. P., Bridge, G. W. K. and Hamilton, M. (1977) The Leeds Scales for the self-assessment of anxiety and depression. *Psychological Test Publications*, Barnstaple.
29. Spielberger, C. D., Gorsuch, R. L. and Lushene, R. E. (1970) *State-trait anxiety inventory manual.* Consulting Psychologists Press, Inc., Palo Alto, California.
30. Watson, D. and Friend, R. (1969) Measurement of social-evaluative anxiety. *Journal of Consulting and Clinical Psychology*, **33**, 448.
31. Locke, H. J. and Wallace, K. M. (1959) Short marital-adjustment and prediction tests: their reliability and validity. *Marriage and Family Living*, p. 251.
32. Dohrenwend, B. P., Shrout, P. E., Egri, G. and Mendelsohn, F. S. (1980) Non-specific psychological distress and other dimensions of psychopathology. *Archives of General Psychiatry*, **37**, 1229.
33. Brown, G. W. and Harris, T. (1978) *Social Origins of Depression*, Tavistock Press, London.
34. Holmes, T. H. and Rahe, R. H. (1967) The social readjustment rating scale. *Journal of Psychosomatic Research*, **11**, 213.

Follow-up of Patients with Inoperable Lung Cancer

J. E. HUGHES

ABSTRACT

Fifty patients with inoperable lung cancer were interviewed by a psychiatrist two to three months after diagnosis. Eight (16%) had a major depressive illness, which was receiving treatment in two cases only. Patients treated by radiotherapy or cytotoxic chemotherapy generally considered treatment worthwhile, whereas patients who had not had active treatment were more likely to be depressed or dissatisfied. Sixteen (32%) would have liked more information about their illness, but twelve (24%) neither knew their diagnosis nor wanted information. Distress among patients' spouses appeared frequent.

This paper presents the results of 50 home interviews with patients suffering from inoperable lung cancer. These interviews were carried out last year, in Southampton, as part of an MRC funded project about the relationship between depression and lung cancer. The interviews were designed to explore three related questions:

1. How common is depressive illness in patients with inoperable lung cancer, and how should it be defined and measured?

These patients have many reasons to be depressed: debilitating physical symptoms, knowledge of having only a short time to live, organic cerebral impairments from complications of their disease. Yet there is no agreed definition of clinical depression in this population. One problem is where to draw the line between appropriate unhappiness and pathological depression. Another problem is the large overlap between the biological symptoms of depressive illness and the symptoms of advanced malignant disease.

2. Is palliative treatment by radiotherapy or cytotoxic drugs worthwhile from most patients' point of view—or are the benefits of these treatments usually outweighed by side-effects, inconvenience, or a sense of futility?
3. Do most patients want to know the facts about their diagnosis and prognosis?

METHOD

Lung cancer had been diagnosed in these patients about three months previously, and they were initially interviewed when first referred to hospital. They had histologically proven lung cancer which was inoperable at presentation. By the time of the three-month follow-up interview, some had completed a course of palliative radiotherapy, some had received several pulses of cytotoxic chemotherapy, and the rest had been allocated to an "observation only" policy. These treatment categories had been decided on ordinary clinical grounds, not in the context of a randomized trial.

A diagnosis of depressive illness was made using a set of symptom criteria obtained at interview. Patients were designated "depressed" if they had at least five of the following symptoms for at least two weeks: depressed mood, tearfulness, loss of interest, poor concentration, irritability, perceiving the illness as a punishment, feelings of guilt or worthlessness, and suicidal thoughts. These criteria resemble the American Psychiatric Association's DSM III criteria for major depression but they exclude the biological symptoms of depression like weight loss, sleep disturbance, and loss of energy, which are impossible to separate from the effects of the cancer itself. They are stringent criteria, only fulfilled by patients with clearcut depressive illness of considerable severity. Milder depression was deliberately excluded as it merges with appropriate reactions to the physical disease.

The interviews also inquired for the following: extent of physical disability using the Karnofsky Scale, patients' opinions of their treatment, patients' knowledge of diagnosis and prognosis, and their satisfaction with the information given by their doctors, and there were some questions about the effect of the illness on patients' marriages, when relevant.

Each interview lasted about half an hour. As many patients were very weak, it was not feasible to explore all potentially relevant topics, and two major omissions were premorbid personality and organic cerebral impairment.

RESULTS

The broad principles of the results are described here, illustrated by some quotations from the interviews, rather than exact figures. A more detailed analysis of these data can be found elsewhere.[1]

The sample consisted of 50 patients, 38 men and 12 women, ranging from 41 to 85 years old. The typical patient was a married man in his sixties who had followed a manual occupation.

Depression

A major depressive illness was present in eight patients: 16% of the sample. To put this finding into perspective: the prevalence of major depressive illness in the general population is between 2% and 5%. Patients with marked physical disability were more likely to be depressed than those who were still active and independent. Depression was also more frequent and severe in patients on "observation only" than in patients on active treatment, although both groups were similar in terms of their levels of physical disability. Age, sex, and marital status were not associated with depression, and the depressed patients were not always the same ones who had been depressed when they initially presented. Two of the eight depressed patients were on tricyclic antidepressants. The other six had apparently not been recognized by their doctors as depressed.

Radiotherapy

Twenty-four patients had received palliative radiotherapy to the chest. None regretted having this treatment. The majority thought it was "definitely" or "probably" worthwhile. "I enjoyed it", "I was disappointed not to get some more." Only three were uncertain, "I know radium won't cure—I don't want to linger on."

The patients' favourable opinions of radiotherapy could not always be explained by lasting relief of physical symptoms, though sometimes this had been achieved. Many patients mentioned other benefits: the kindness of radiotherapy staff, their satisfaction on "having something done".

Half the radiotherapy patients reported no adverse side-effects at all: "Nothing to it" was a repeated comment. Others, given identical treatment regimes, reported almost intolerable side effects: "Very hard to cope with—it shattered me."

Inquiries about the most unpleasant side effect revealed physical and emotional malaise, shortly after each treatment, to be top of the list.

Chemotherapy

Fifteen patients with oat cell tumours were having combination chemotherapy with cyclophosphamide, adriamycin and VP16. Their opinions resembled those from the radiotherapy group, though chemotherapy was not regarded quite so favourably as radiotherapy, and more often caused troublesome side effects.

Again, no patient regretted having chemotherapy. Most chemotherapy patients thought treatment was worthwhile: "It's not pleasant for the first week, but then you get two good weeks and that's not so bad, considering what's wrong." Three were uncertain—"It's worthwhile if it's doing me good and I can't say if it is or not." Again, kindness of staff was much appreciated. Patients having chemotherapy usually seemed well informed about their illness, with a sense of participation in treatment decisions, which was also appreciated. Nausea and vomiting topped the list of "worst side effects". Though hair loss affected all patients, only one woman said it caused her severe distress.

Observation only

The eleven observation only patients included three who were profoundly depressed. All three had experienced a physical deterioration since their last hospital visit, were having uncontrolled pain, and suspected they had cancer but had not been told. "They say it's not conclusive what's wrong and I needn't go back for three months—but I'm afraid I'll have gone so far downhill by then they won't be able to do anything." "They've talked to me but in essence told me nothing—it's my belief I've reached the final chapter of my life." Three others were puzzled and rather discontent, though not formally depressed, whereas the other five showed no distress. One man said "I was very pleased I didn't need treatment—I don't like hospitals."

Knowledge of Diagnosis and Prognosis

No cases of depression were found among the patients who did not seem to have any idea they had cancer, nor among those who believed they would recover. However, depression was more frequent among those who suspected their diagnosis than those who had it openly confirmed.

Thirty patients expressed complete satisfaction with the information their doctors had given them. This group included twelve who had apparently not been given any information at all—three of them emphasized they did not want any. Sixteen patients would have liked to know more about their illness. Most of them said they had not liked to ask questions: "I didn't want to waste their time with all the others queuing up outside", "It's not my place to ask, they decide what you should know." Two patients had asked direct questions but had not received truthful answers: "I asked what the biopsy showed but he said the lab had lost it." "He said we don't know what's wrong but at least it's not cancer."

No patient said they had been told too much or regretted knowing their diagnosis. Many were relieved when their suspicions of cancer were confirmed: "I was pleased to know what I'd got to fight against." "I was pleased when he told me—at least there was no more question of malingering."

Spouses' Reactions

Thirty-six patients were married at the time of interview. Half of them unreservedly praised their wife or husband for their support: wives were described as "excellent", "an angel", "a godsend". The rest were concerned by their spouse's distress. "She's got so poorly and run down, I'm afraid my cough keeps her awake at night." A few patients perceived themselves as the "coping" partner who was having to look after a spouse overwhelmed with anxiety or grief.

Twenty-six married patients knew their diagnosis and ten of these could not discuss it freely with their spouse. "I try to talk to him but he gets so terribly upset. He wants to hide his head in the sand." Two patients' wives described the strain experienced because they had been told their husband's diagnosis whereas he had not.

COMMENTS AND CONCLUSIONS

Severe depression affects a substantial number of lung cancer patients—16% in this study—but apparently often goes unremarked. This may be because of problems in diagnosis, or because it is considered an understandable response to the disease, or because many of the patients concerned are diffident and unable to express their problems. Severe depression may be equally common in these patients' husbands and wives.

Confident comparisons cannot be made between treatment groups, as allocation was not random and numbers in each group were small, but morale seems better among patients given palliative radiotherapy or chemotherapy than among those given no active treatment. This is not always because palliative treatment prevents a deterioration in physical state: rather, I think, it is because an "observation-only" policy often means less frequent doctor–patient contact, so less efficient detection of physical or mental problems, and less readiness to answer patients' questions frankly. Perhaps doctors are especially likely to avoid the difficult task of conveying a diagnosis of advanced lung cancer when they are unable to temper the bad news with an offer of active treatment.

A minority of patients were happy to remain ignorant of their diagnosis and prognosis. Most, however, preferred to know the truth. Poor communication between patient and doctor, and between patient and spouse, was a common problem which seemed to have a link with depressive states.

So, how should depression occurring in association with lung cancer be managed? From the evidence presented here, I believe the problem could be reduced by more attention to good doctor–patient relationships, but this will not always be sufficient. We do not know the efficacy of antidepressant drugs or ECT in this population, and more research is needed here.

REFERENCE

1. Hughes, J. E. (1985) Depressive illness and lung cancer II: Follow-up of inoperable patients. *European Journal of Surgical Oncology*, **11**, 21–24.

Coping with Cancer:
The Positive Approach

T. MORRIS

ABSTRACT

In what way might attitudes towards a diagnosis of cancer influence survival? Are certain early attitudes to diagnosis favourable for later psychological adjustment? Should the "confronting" approaches advocated by some alternative medicine practitioners be incorporated into routine care of cancer patients?

A method for rating responses to the idea of "having cancer" has been developed using semi-structured interviews from 170 breast cancer and lymphoma patients to derive patients' cognitive responses.

Three types of responses are described: appraisals and palliating and confronting strategies. The majority of patients use palliating strategies; only half the patient sample use any confronting strategies. These patients use more strategies overall, they feel more in control of their health and, one year following diagnosis, they tend to be less depressed and anxious.

Particular strategies associated with lower depression and anxiety scores at 3 and 12 months post-diagnosis suggest that a policy of "selective ignoring", leaving the medical problem to someone else and making positive plans works best; in addition, at 3 months only, limiting objectives and reflecting that others share one's predicament are effective. This latter finding could have implications for management.

Is it beneficial for patients to adopt a confronting attitude to their cancer diagnosis; to change their thinking and behaviour, to marshall their mental and physical resources in an attempt to increase their length of survival? Alternative therapies, based on this notion, have grown up in the United Kingdom[1] and elsewhere,[2, 3] despite the fact that studies in this area do not show a consistent pattern of results.

At least one aim of research in this area, carried out during the last three years in the Faith Courtauld Unit, has been to develop a method for recording attitudes to cancer diagnosis so that they might be described and any association between particular attitudes and survival documented.[4] Now that such a method has been developed, it is possible to describe the patterns of attitudes and cognitive strategies we observed in our patient sample; and also to see whether any of these attitudes and strategies were associated with lower levels of psychological morbidity on various outcome measures.

METHOD

Measures of Attitude to Cancer

Cognitive strategies

These responses are mental devices by means of which patients appeared to manipulate their *thinking* about "having cancer". Two were used:
  (i) P: *Palliating strategies* are those by means of which patients try to *reduce* the mental impact of having cancer, e.g. "trying not to think about it".
  (ii) C: *Confronting strategies* are ways by means of which patients try to encourage themselves to think positively about their lives without in any way trying to mitigate the potential harm associated with a cancer diagnosis, e.g. "planning enjoyable activities".

Behaviour

Patients reported various actions that they had taken as a result of cancer diagnosis and treatment which we categorized into 21 different behaviours, e.g. "distracting himself with activities", "avoiding people", "practising alternative therapy".

Features of the style of the interview

We also made observations on the verbal characteristics and content of the interviews.[4]

Locus of Control

Patients also completed the Health Locus of Control Scales[5] in order to determine how far they felt able to control their health.

Measures of Emotional Distress[4]

The Wakefield Depression Inventory[6] and the Spielberger State-Trait Anxiety Inventory[7] were used as "outcome measures" of the effectiveness of the cognitive strategies.

Sample

A series of 108 breast cancer and 62 male and female lymphoma patients were interviewed 3 and 12 months post-diagnosis.[4]

RESULTS

Whereas the great majority of patients described palliating strategies which they used, more than half of the patients, male and female, breast cancer and lymphoma, used no confronting strategies at all (82 vs. 77). It was thus likely that there were differences on other variables between patients who used confronting responses and those who did not. Comparisons between patients who used confronting strategies versus those who did not revealed a number of significant differences between these two groups.

Patients who reported using confronting strategies also used significantly more palliating strategies (4.2 vs. 3.1, $p > 0.001$). They reported more behaviours (2.9 vs. 2.4, $p > 0.05$) and they had higher scores on the Internal Health Locus of Control Scale[7] (25.7 vs. 23.9, $p > 0.05$), that is they felt they had more control over their health. There were tendencies, too, for them to have lower scores on the Wakefield Depression Inventory (8.4 vs. 10.3, $p = 0.07$); and on the Trait measure of the Spielberger Anxiety Inventory, than their non-confronting counterparts (34.5 vs. 37.1, $p = 0.10$). Finally, there was a tendency for those who used confronting strategies, 3 months post-diagnosis, to be less depressed (7.7 vs. 9.7, p = 0.07) and less anxious (33.7 vs. 35.7, p = 0.20) 12 months after diagnosis.

Since most patients used Palliating strategies, we divided them into high P and low P responders. Depression scores tended to be lower (7.8 vs. 9.6, p = 0.10) at 12 months, but anxiety scores were significantly lower in those using a large number of Palliating strategies (33.1 vs. 36.3, p = 0.05). This finding supports our hypothesis that these strategies are developed as a means of reducing anxiety.

These results suggest that a combination of Palliating and Confronting strategies, in other words a flexible approach to the problem of managing the emotional response to cancer diagnosis, could be effective in reducing mood disturbance on the outcome measures at 12 months. This hypothesis was tested by separately correlating the total number of Palliating and Confronting strategies with the outcome measures. There was a small but significant negative correlation between the *total* number of Palliating and Confronting strategies and both the Wakefield Depression Inventory (r = −0.16, p < 0.05, n = 135) and the Spielberger Anxiety Inventory (r = −0.17, p < 0.01, n = 135). These results are, however, almost entirely accounted for by the total number of Palliating strategies since the values for Confronting strategies and for the Wakefield and Spielberger Inventories are very low (r = −0.10 and −0.05 respectively). Thus it seems that Palliating strategies may play a larger part in reducing depression and anxiety scores one year following diagnosis than do Confronting strategies. It is important to note, however, that these data are for the *whole sample*, and that there may be differences between males and females, breast cancer and lymphoma patients, and those who have recurrence compared with those who do not.

To determine whether any particular factors might be associated with scores on measures of anxiety and depression, individual Palliating and Confronting strategies, reported behaviours and features of the style of the interview were also correlated with Wakefield and Spielberger Scores at 3 and 12 months post-diagnosis. Factors associated with lower depression and anxiety scores at 3 and 12 months are listed in Tables 1 and 2. The lists suggest the different nature of the coping task for patients at 3 and at 12 months post-diagnosis. At 3 months, it seems that patients who have lower depression scores are concerned with not being too ambitious in their goals ("limiting objectives"), reflecting that they are not alone ("reflecting that others share predicament") and are helped by the concern that others show for them ("incorporating others' exhortations"); whereas at 12 months, rather than reflecting on a predicament shared with others, those with lower mood disturbance scores "avoid reminders of the diagnosis". At *both* time points, a favourable outcome is associated with a sense that the *disease* outcome is not something that the patient feels responsible for ("outcome lies in the hands of others") and an ability to turn the mind to "making life enjoyable". At 12 months, to this latter strategy has been added a strategy which displays an orientation to the future, that is "planning positive activities".

TABLE 1. FACTORS ASSOCIATED WITH LOWER DEPRESSION SCORES

		At three months
P	3_4	Limiting objectives
P	4_1	Outcome lies in the hands of others
P	9_1	Concentrating on making life enjoyable
P	9_4	Reflecting that others share predicament
C	2_2	Incorporating others' exhortations
		Lower anxiety scores
P	5_2	Emphasizing others' concern for patient

TABLE 2. FACTORS ASSOCIATED WITH LOWER DEPRESSION SCORES

		At twelve months
P	4_1	Outcome lies in the hands of others
P	9_1	Concentrating on making life enjoyable
P	9_2	Concentrating on mitigating aspects of disease
C	5	Planning positive activities
D	20	Avoiding reminders of diagnosis
		Lower anxiety scores
P	5_2	Emphasizing others' concern for patient

By contrast, those with high mood disturbance scores at 3 and 12 months display little ability to manage emotional distress at the cognitive level (Tables 3 and 4). At 3-month interviews, these individuals were often visibly emotionally distressed. They described themselves as experiencing outbursts of intense emotion, trying to distract themselves, avoiding sympathetic approaches by others and trying not to think about their disease. At 12 months, individuals who are distressed again demonstrate how few intrapsychic capacities they have for coping with distress. The

T. Morris

picture is of an individual whose only responses are "trying not to think about the problem", "seeking information" (perhaps on which to base a strategy for the management of emotional distress) and "cutting down obligations" in an attempt to reduce the demands upon him or her.

TABLE 3. FACTORS ASSOCIATED WITH HIGHER DEPRESSION SCORES

		At three months
E	1	General dissatisfaction with life
E	4	Emotive outpourings in interview
E	8	Overexpansion of account
D	1	Intense emotional outbursts
D	18	Distracting himself
D	21	Avoiding others' sympathy
		Higher anxiety scores
P	1	Trying not to think about it

TABLE 4. FACTORS ASSOCIATED WITH HIGHER DEPRESSION SCORES

		At twelve months
P	1_1	Trying not to think about it
E	1	General dissatisfaction with life
D	13	Seeking information
		Higher anxiety scores
D	24	Cutting down obligations

DISCUSSION

The central role of cognition in assuaging emotional pain is demonstrated by the contrast in the responses of patients with high and low mood disturbance 12 months after cancer diagnosis. In the highly distressed, there is an *absence* of cognitive strategies suggesting that the individual is able only to try to shut out painful emotions by not thinking them, leading to higher, rather than lower, levels of anxiety. The data suggest that distressed individuals are experiencing a failure of cognitive control.

It is striking that, far from adopting confronting attitudes, those who have low levels of anxiety and depression adopt a strategy of "selective ignoring". They do not attempt to change those aspects of the disease which may not lie within the individual's control; rather, they concentrate on making life enjoyable.

REFERENCES

1. Forbes, A. (1981) Cancer and its non-toxic treatment: working your way back to health. Privately published.
2. Simonton, O. C., M-Simonton, S. and Geighton, J. (1978) *Getting Well Again.* J. P. Tarcher, Los Angeles.
3. Meares, A. (1979) Meditation: a psychological approach to cancer treatment. *Practitioner,* **222,** 119–122.
4. Morris, T., Blake, S. and Buckley, M. (1985) Development of a method for rating cognitive responses to a diagnosis of cancer. *Social Science and Medicine,* **8,** 795–802.
5. Wallston, K. A., Wallston, B. S. and DeVellis, R. (1978) Development of the multidimensional health locus of control scale (M.H.L.C.). *Health Education Monographs,* **6,** 160–170.
6. Snaith, R. P., Ahmed, S. N., Mehta, S. and Hamilton, M. (1971) Assessment of the severity of primary depressive illness. *Psychological Medicine,* **1,** 143–149.
7. Spielberger, C. D., Gorsuch, R. C. and Lushene, R. E. (1970) *The State-Trait Anxiety Inventory.* Consulting Psychologists Press, Palo Alto, California.

Coping with Hodgkin's Disease and Non-Hodgkin's Lymphoma

J. DEVLEN

ABSTRACT

A prospective study has confirmed that the diagnosis and treatment of Hodgkin's disease and non-Hodgkin's lymphoma is associated with considerable psychiatric morbidity and treatment toxicity. Of the 120 patients followed up for twelve months from diagnosis, 23% suffered an anxiety state and 22% developed a depressive illness. Nausea, vomiting, hair loss, a sore mouth and changes in taste were the most commonly experienced side effects of treatment. A method of assessing patients' concerns and coping strategies was developed during the study. This classification of coping was described and some preliminary results presented of patients' concerns, their coping strategies and how these might be related to psychological outcome.

87

Index